How to Grow Medical Marijuana: An in-Depth Quick Grow Guide: with over 155 photos/illustrations

By David Curran

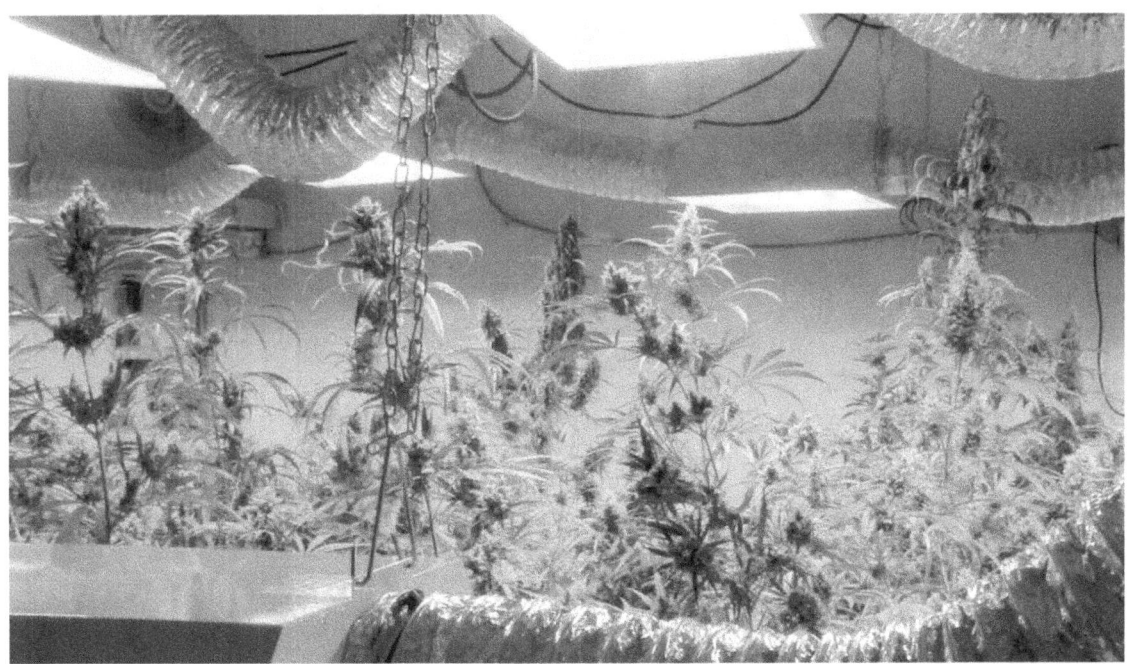

Most medical marijuana patients don't have the kind of room it takes to grow huge plants the way this operation does.

What they might have is room for two small grow rooms, like the ones I'll show you here which measure 2 x 2 x 6.

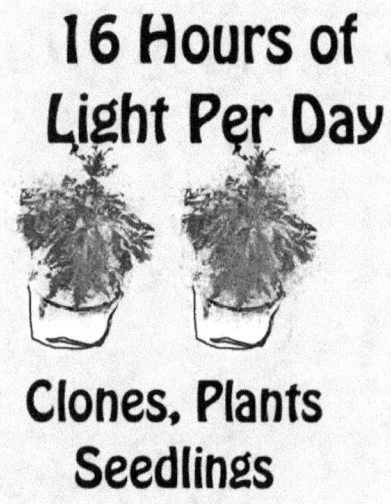

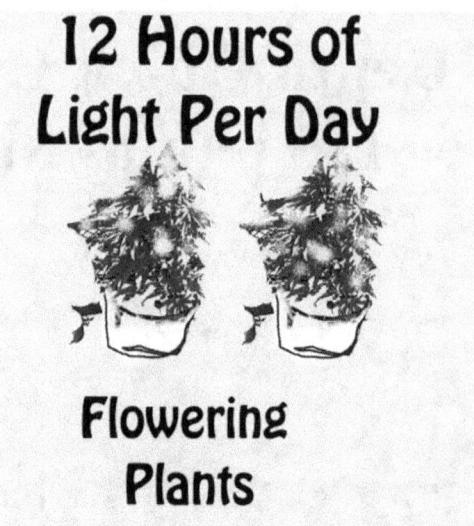

You'll need two separate areas for your grow sheds because although Clones, Seedlings and growing plants can do well on 16 hours per day, flowering plants need a full 12 hours of darkness to flower and produce medicine.

Now some of you may have heard that some growers keep the lights on in their grow room for 24 hours a day. I recommend 16 hours a day, because I grow from feminized seed and female clones and increased light can cause a female plant to produce male flowers. We don't want male flowers in our bloom shed because unfertilized females produce more medicine.

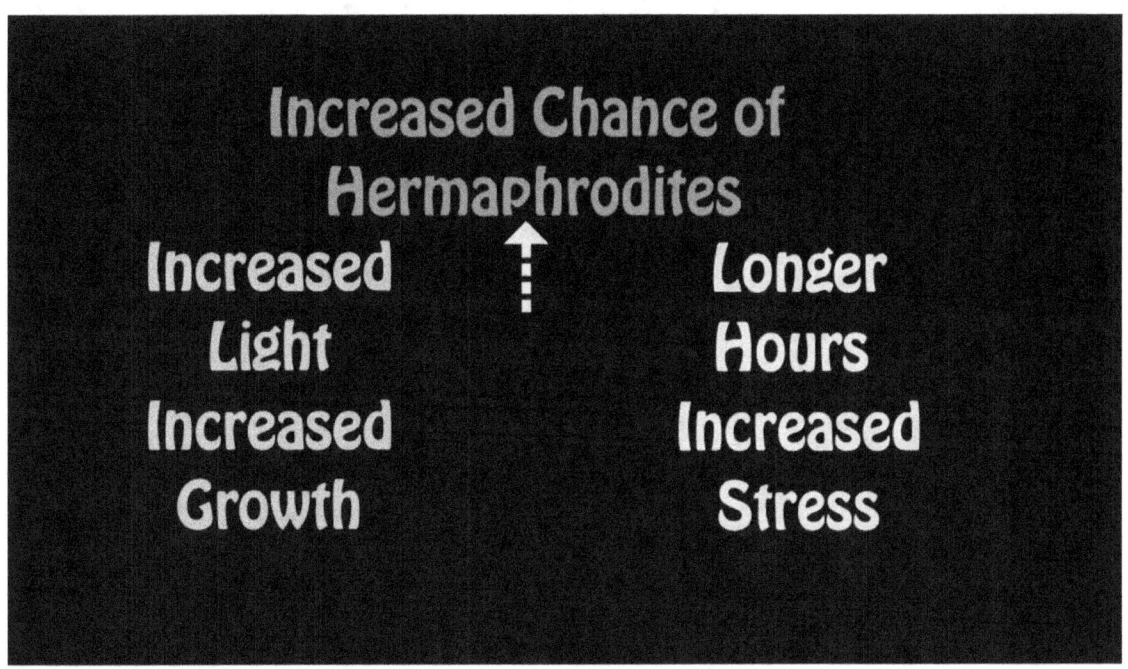

For our grow sheds we chose plastic sheds since the humidity in a grow shed can cause damage to wood.

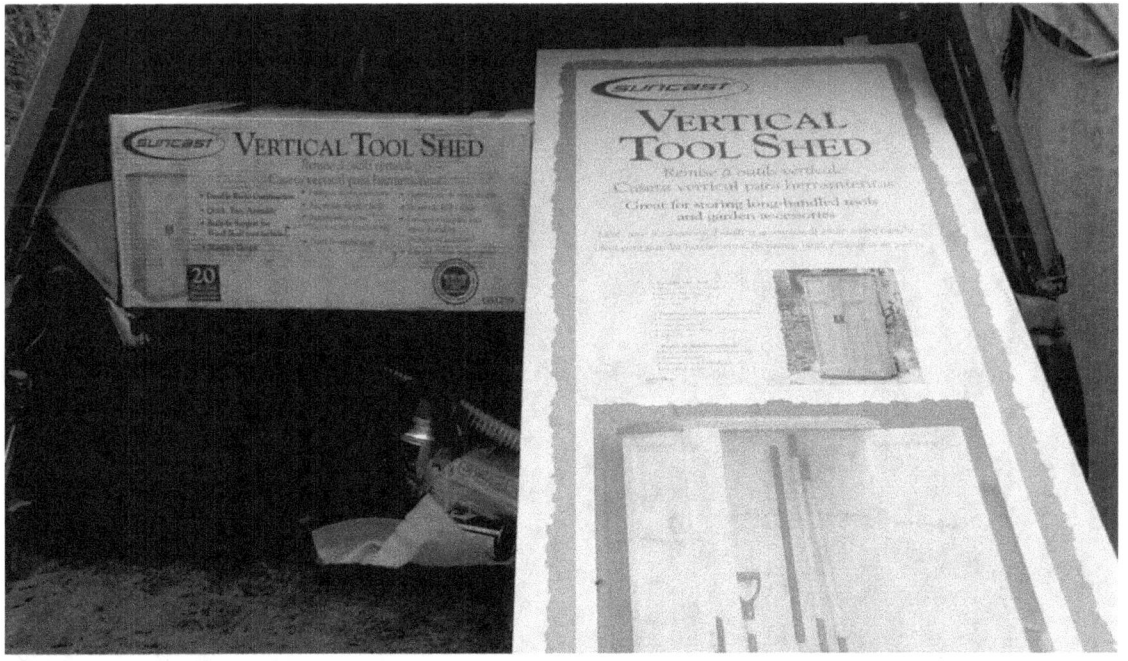

You will need duct hose and pipe from various hardware stores. This will be used to vent your sheds and provide air-flow. (Photos of completed shed follow.)

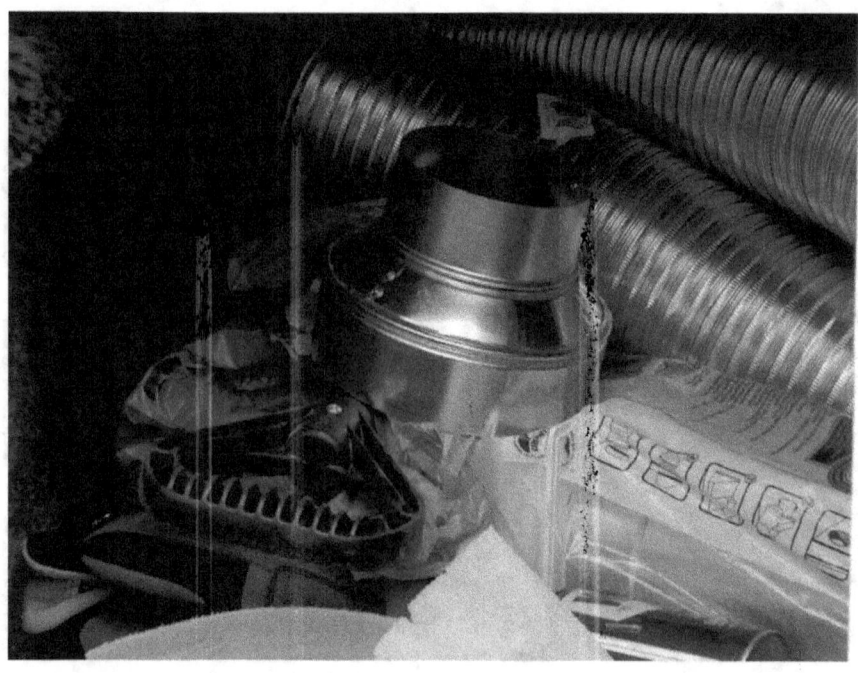

For paint we chose a latex primer. Most white paints these days are not really 'flat' and primer was actually flatter. If I had it to do it over I would have used an oil-based primer.

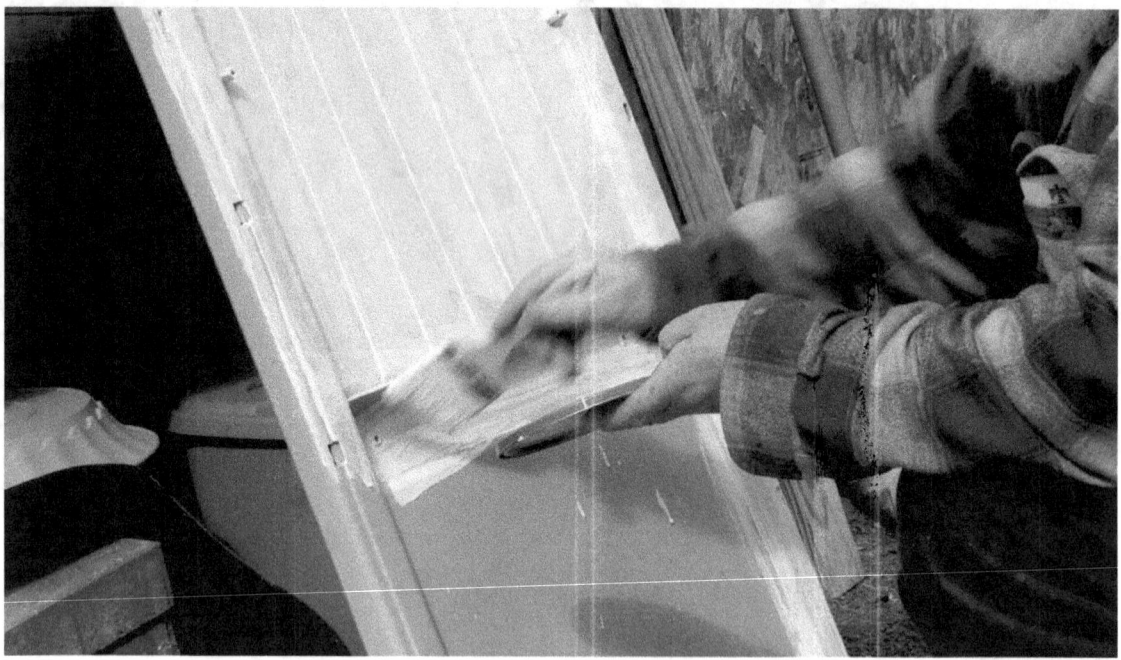

One gallon was more than enough for the two sheds with three coats each.

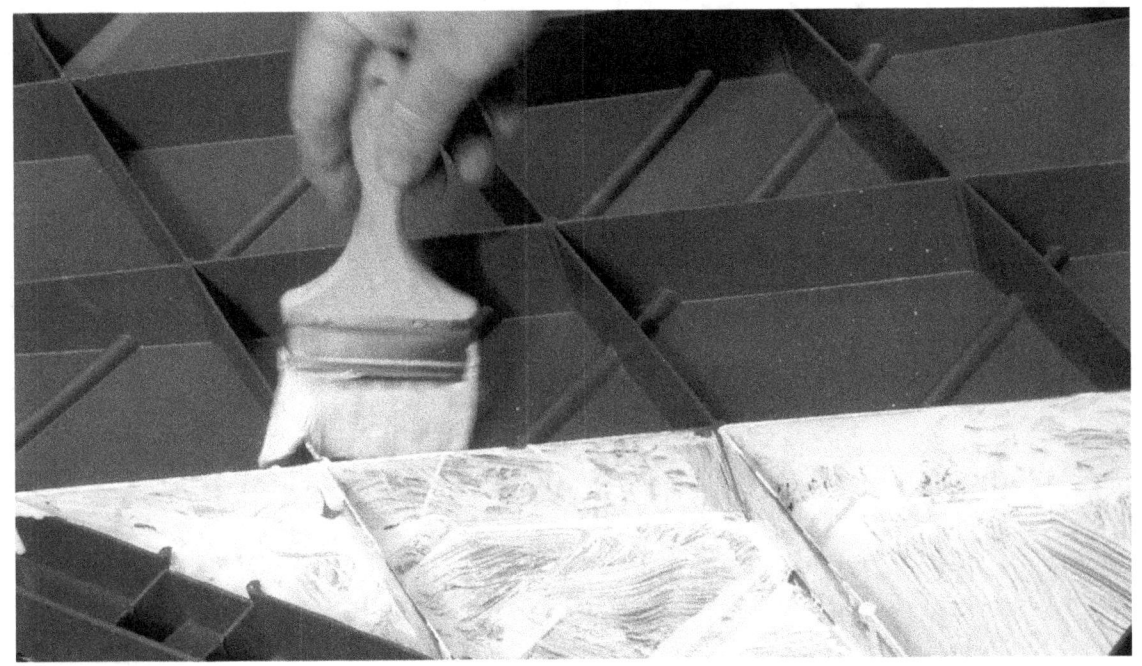

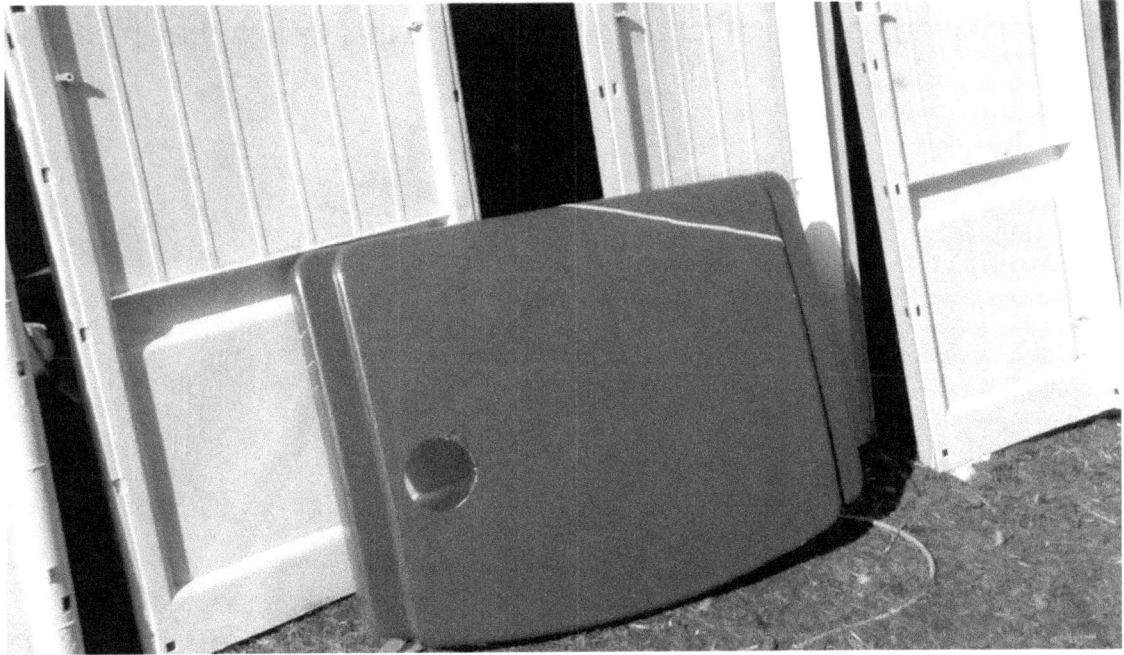

We let each coat dry before applying the next.

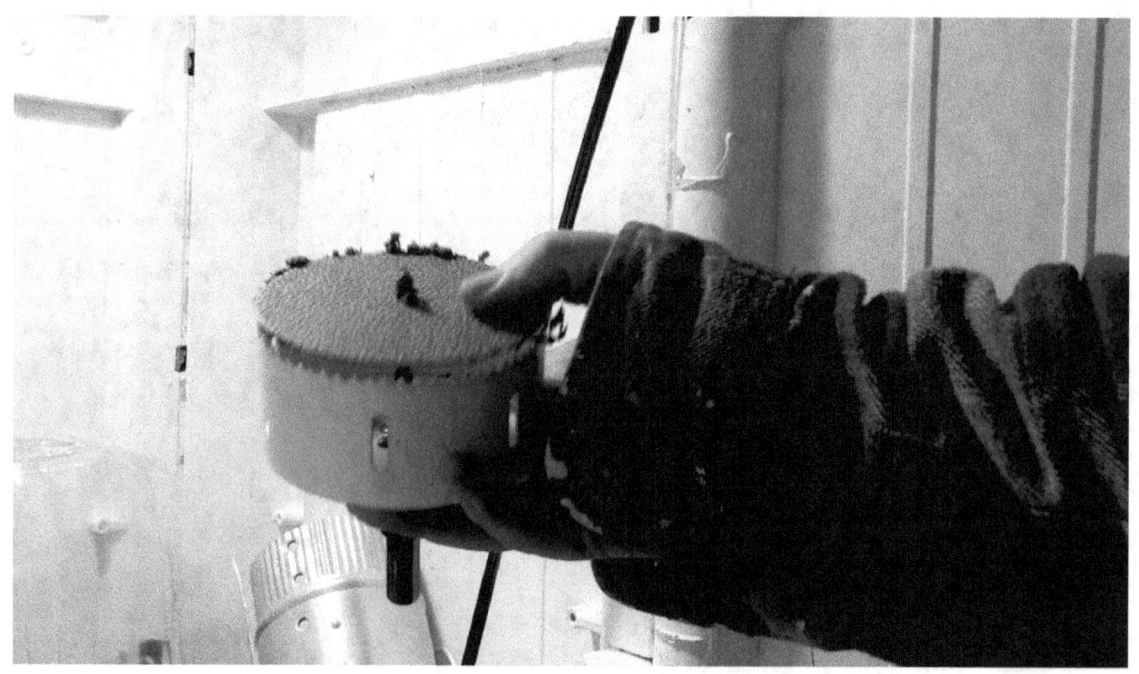

A four inch drill bit is perfect for cutting a hole that 4-inch duct pipe will fit.

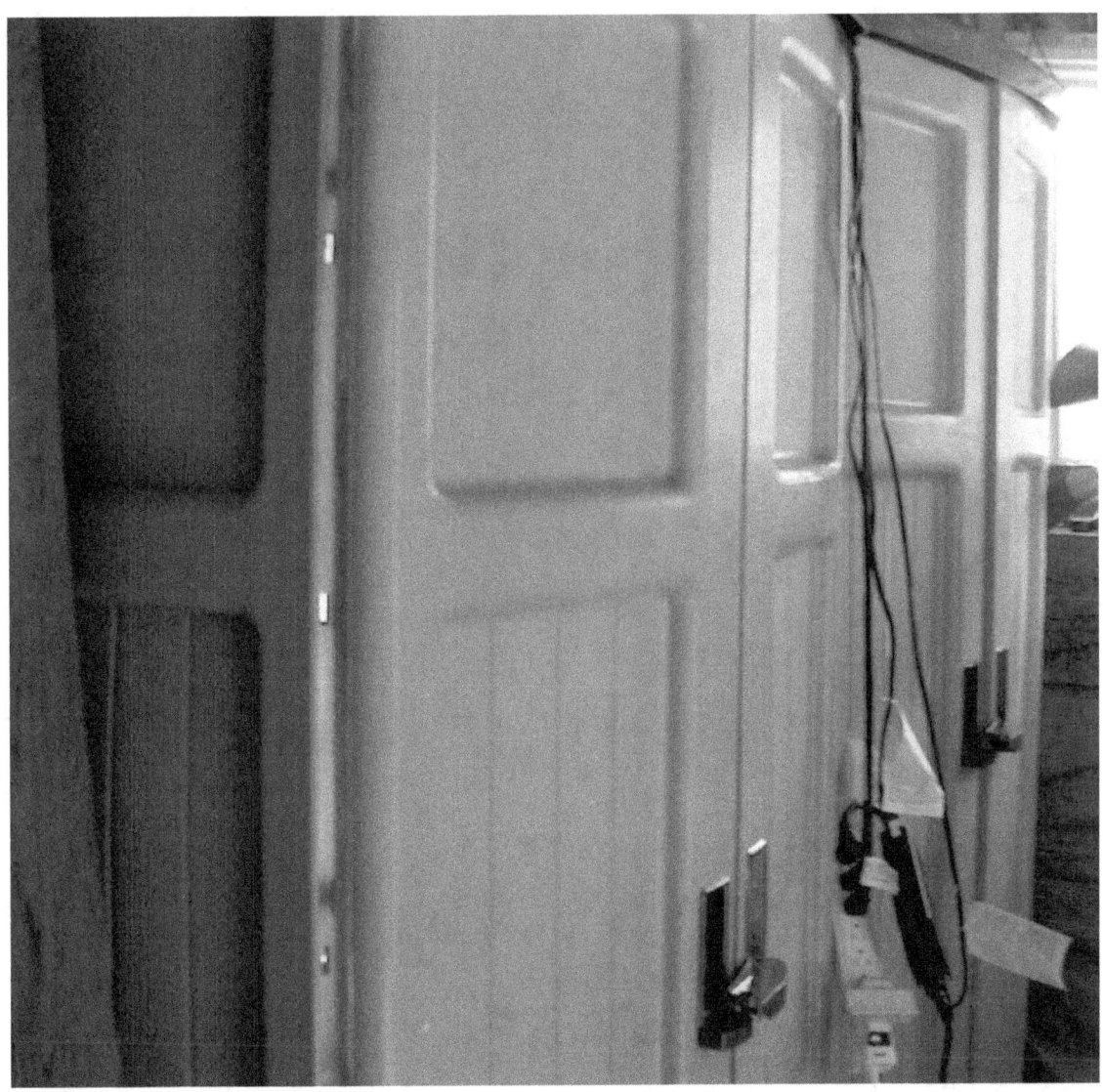

Side by side the cabinets don't take up too much room. You could use any cabinets available as long as you have the space inside.

The set-up I use is one 80 Cubic feet per minute vent fan per shed, and one 250 CFM fan that works with both sheds. The vents and fans provide much needed air to the plants and also help control temperature in the sheds.

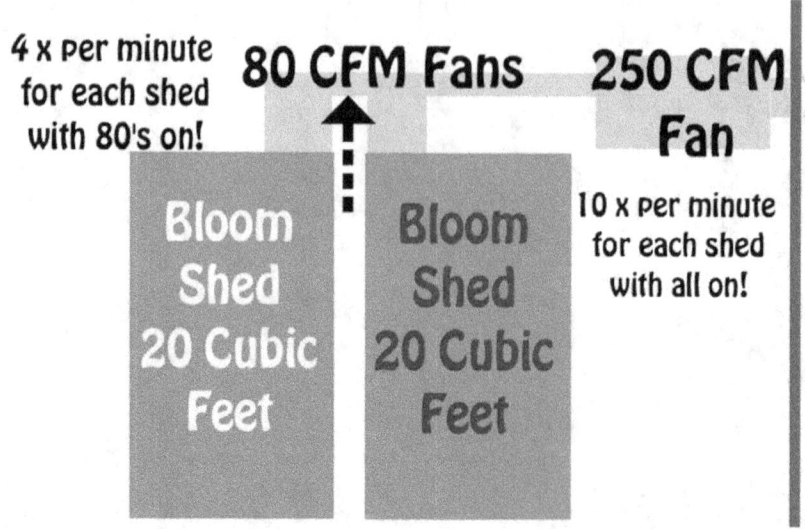

4 x per minute for each shed with 80's on! **80 CFM Fans** **250 CFM Fan**

Bloom Shed 20 Cubic Feet **Bloom Shed 20 Cubic Feet** **10 x per minute for each shed with all on!**

Another reason for the ventilation is that in combination with a humidifier it can control the temperature of our shed.

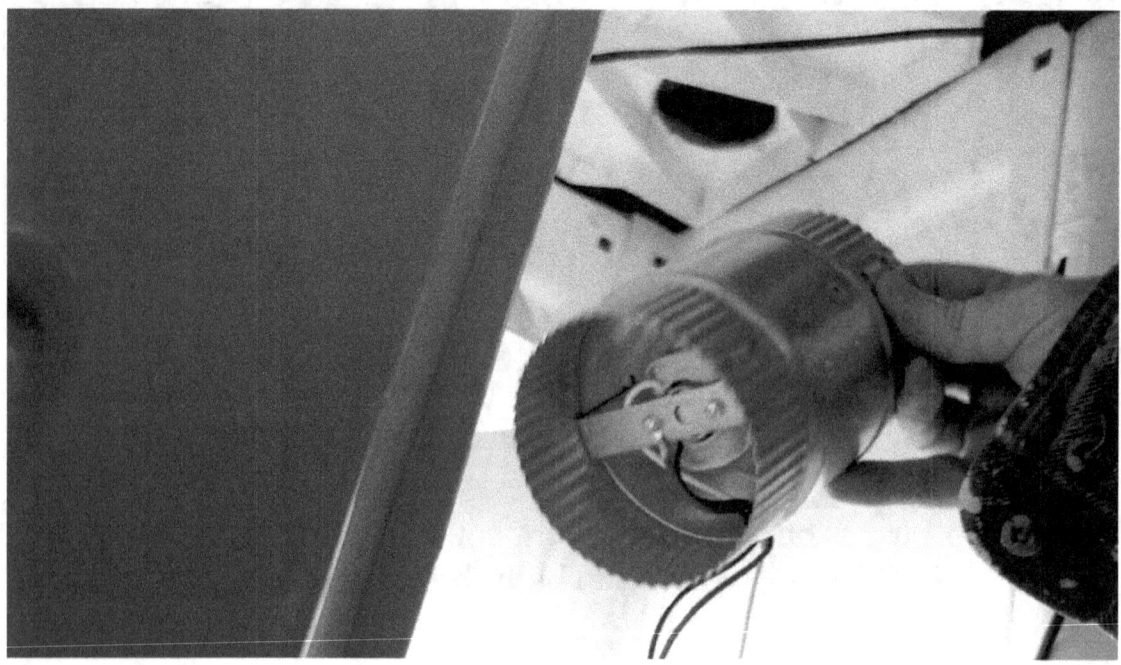

In line fans are not very expensive and made to operate for a long time quietly.

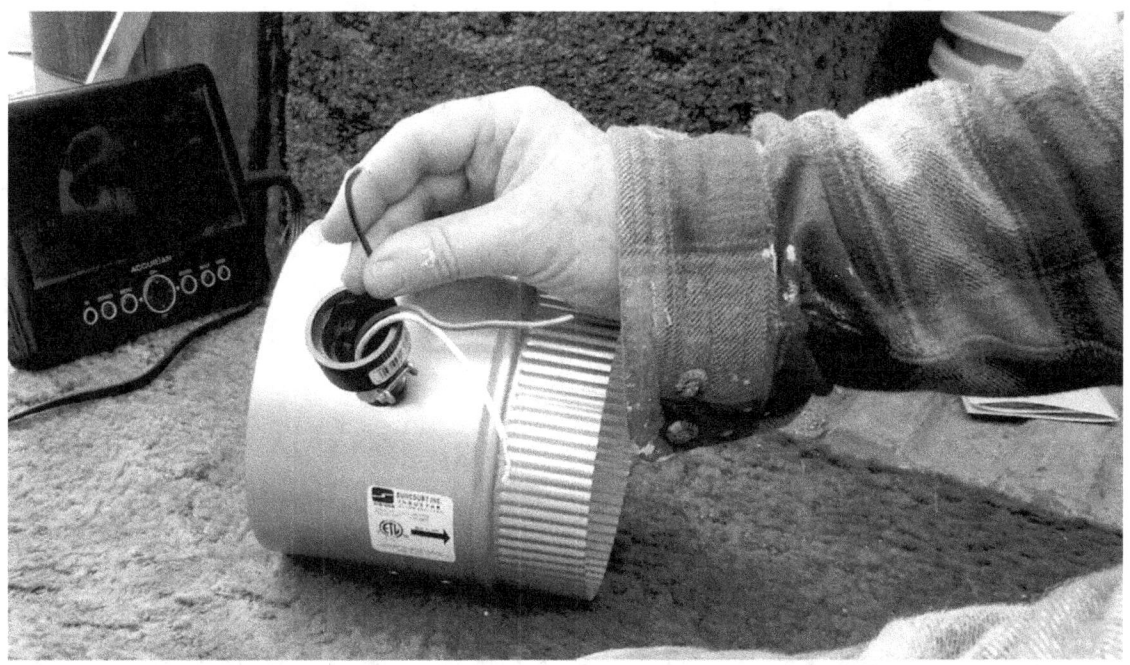

They usually come without plugs because they are often connected to temperature or humidity controls. For my purposes, I intended to run them all day, I needed to add plugs.

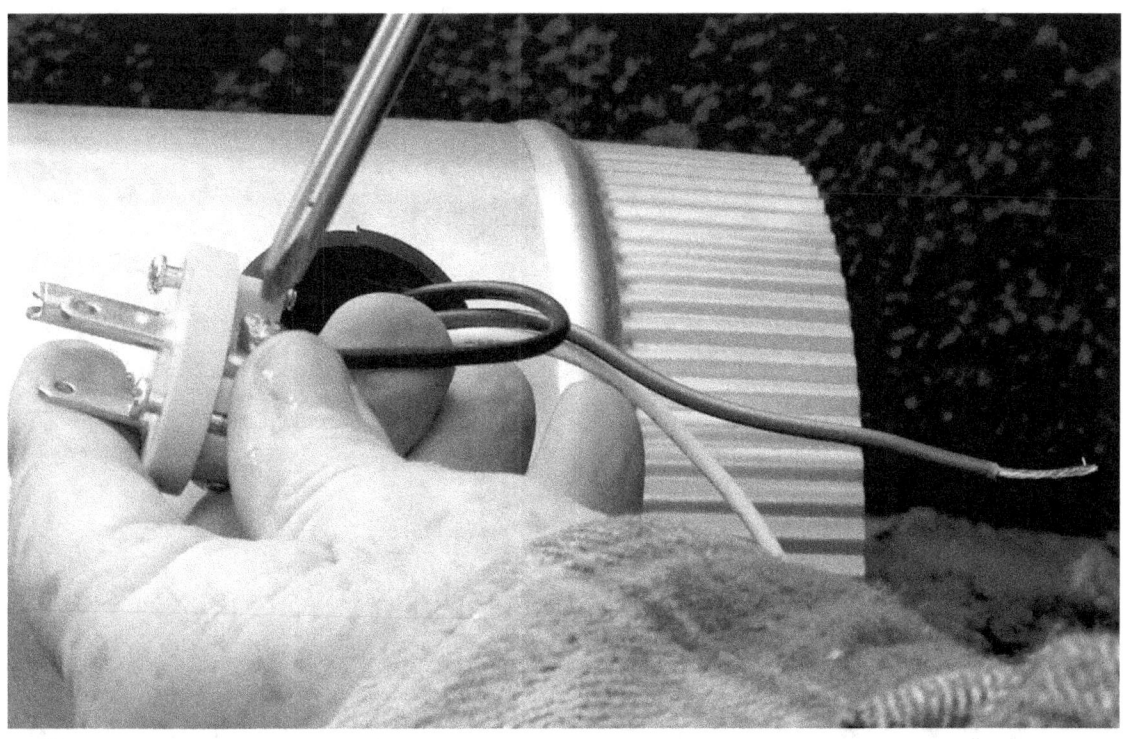

Installation is simple. Black goes to the brass screw, white to the sliver screw and the groun --the green or bare copper wire---goes to the green screw.

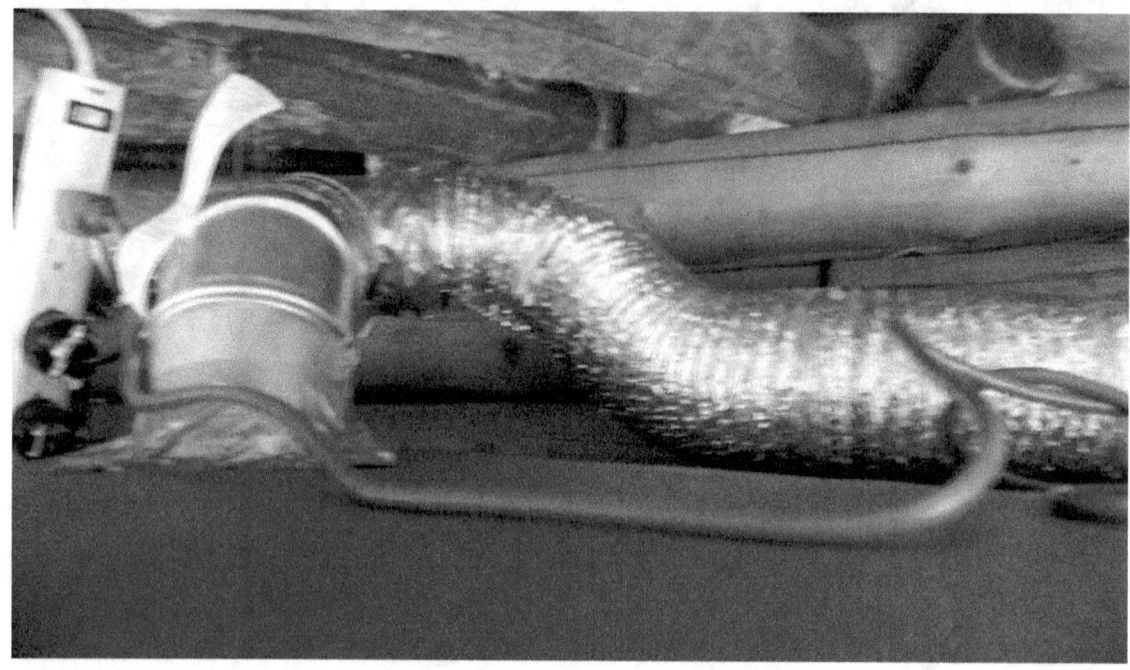

Setup was easy. I used metal tighteners to attach the hose to the pipe and duct tape on pipe to pipe connections.

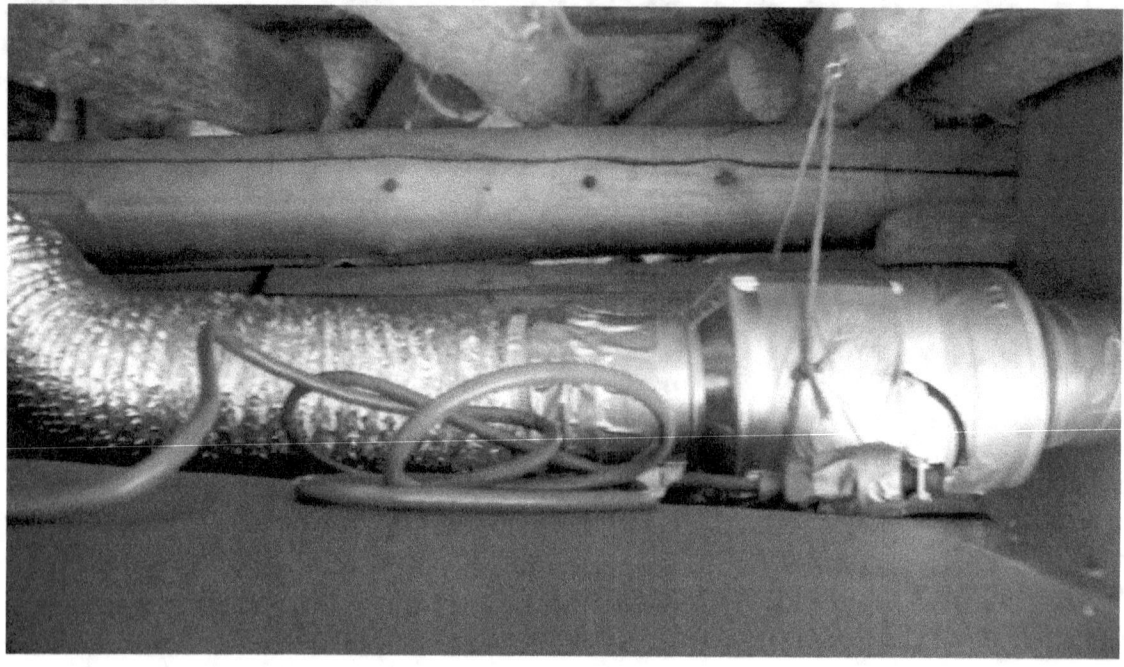

Make sure you have all the adapters you need. I forgot one 6"
connector and had to use duct tape and ice cream sticks to modify.

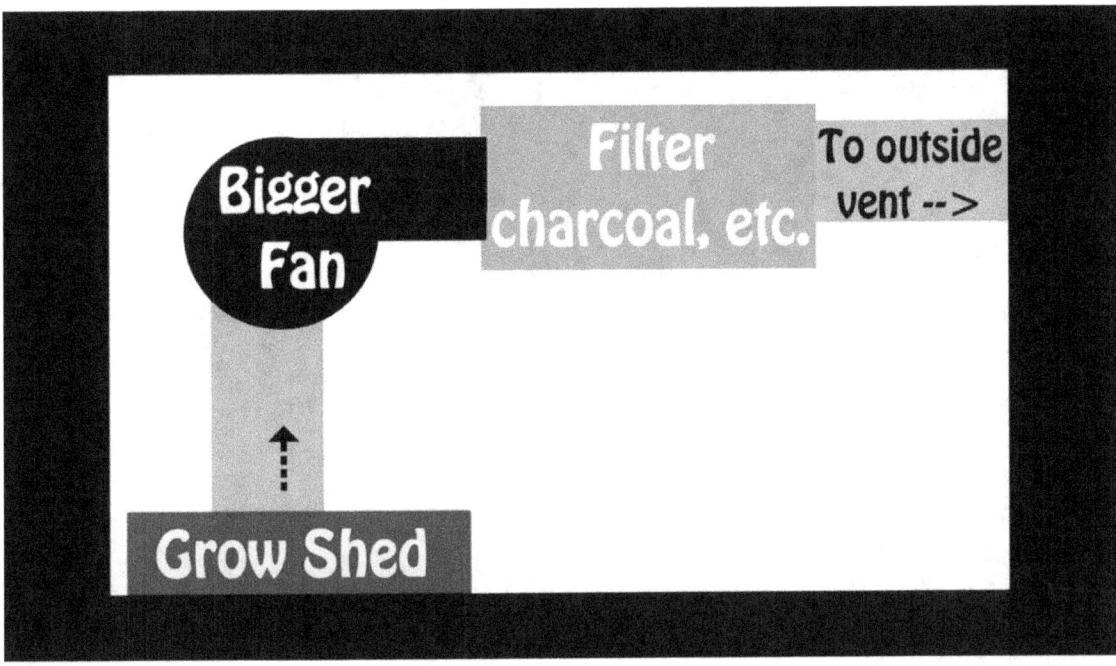

If you are growing medical marijuana with a permit you may not have to
worry about the smell. But if it is a problem a charcoal filter will reduce
the problem. Keep in mind you may need a much more powerful fan
than our little in-line duct fans to push air through a filter.

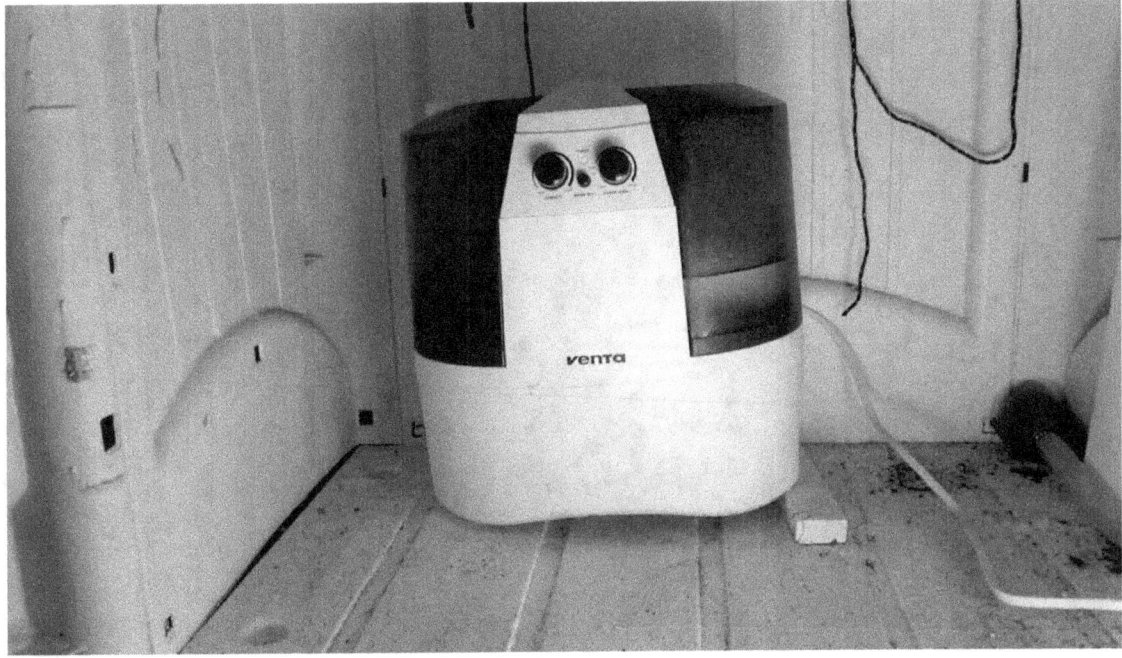

To control humidity for clones just coming out of a humidity dome, or young plants, I use a Venta Sonic humidifier.

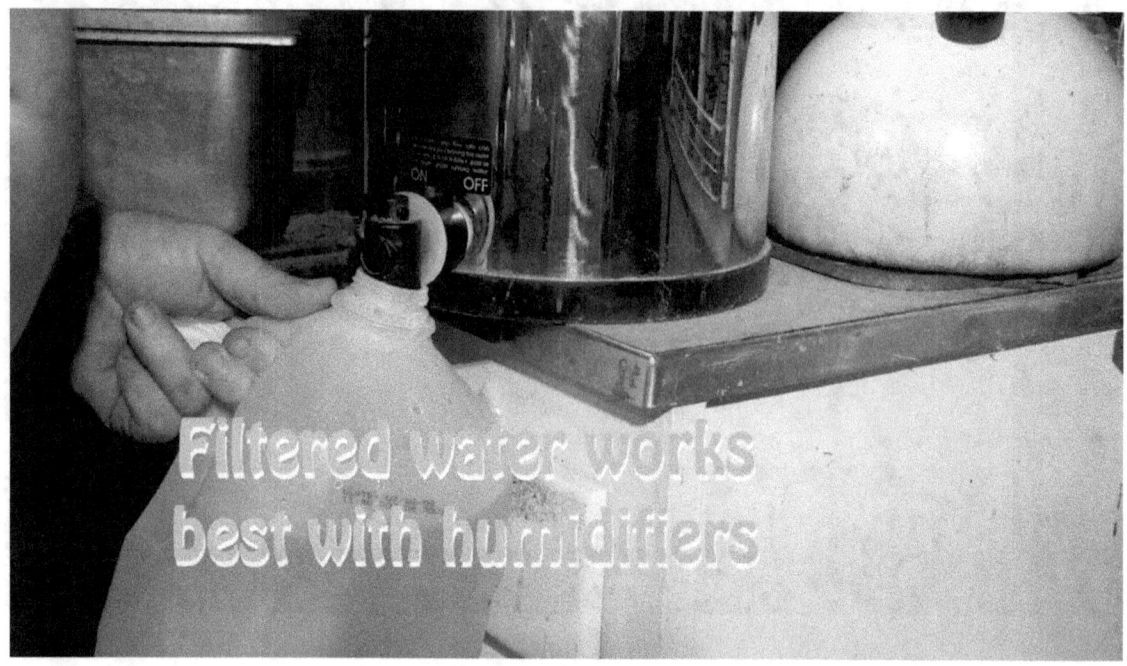

Humidifiers work better with filtered water.

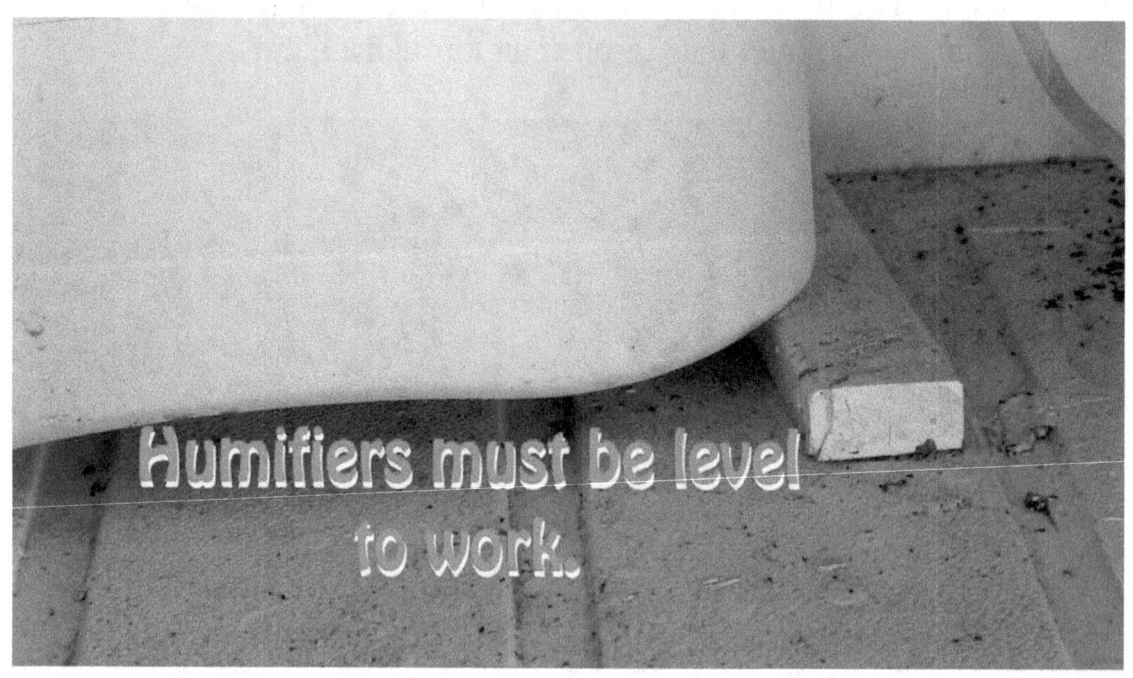

More expensive humidifiers sense when they are off balance and shut down. You'll have to have your humidifier level for it to work properly.

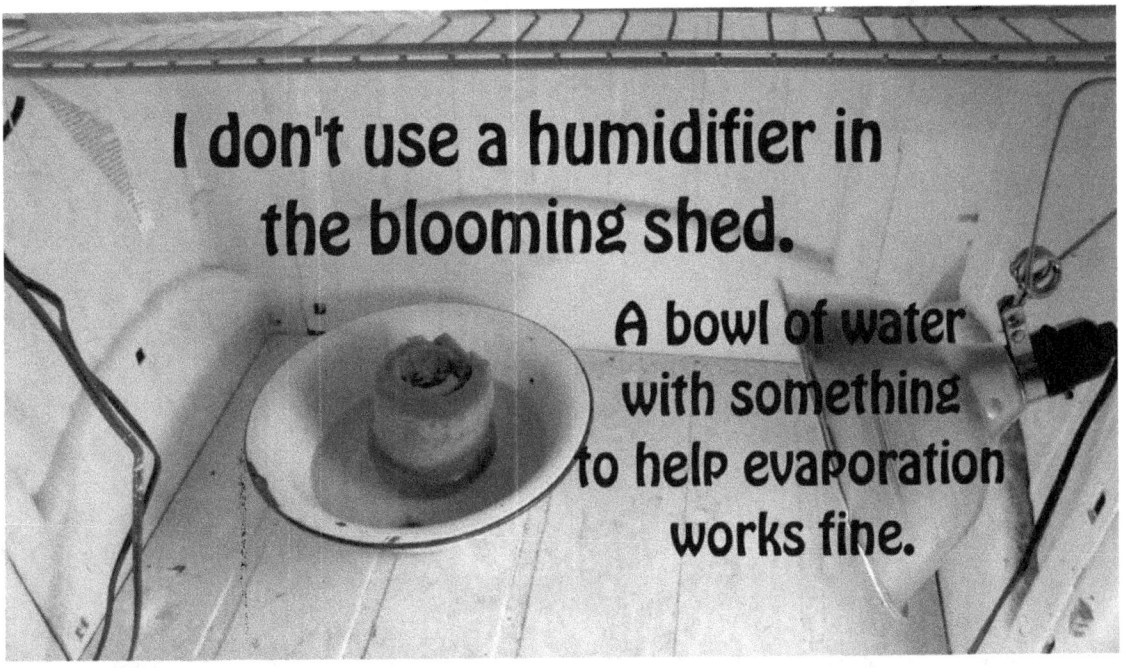

An alternative to a humidifier can be a bowl of water with something to help evaporate the water. A fan on the bowl can put even more moisture into the air.

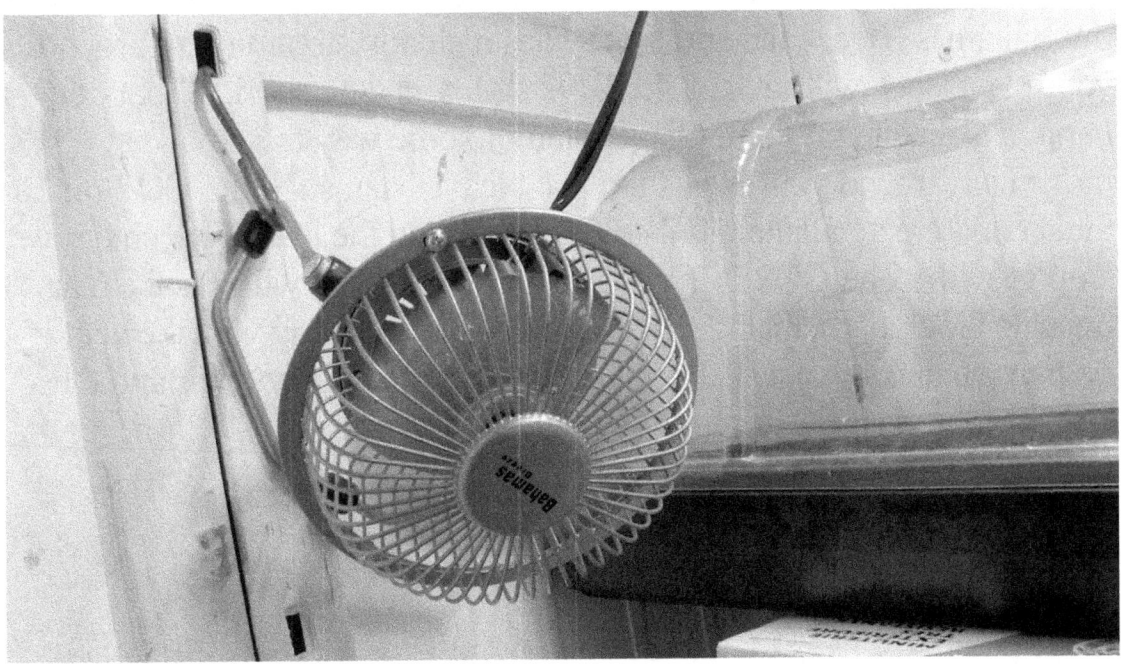

When I started out I used larger fans—actually old ones I had on hand. But I found this tiny Bahamas Breeze fans used less power but put a steady stream of air over my plants.

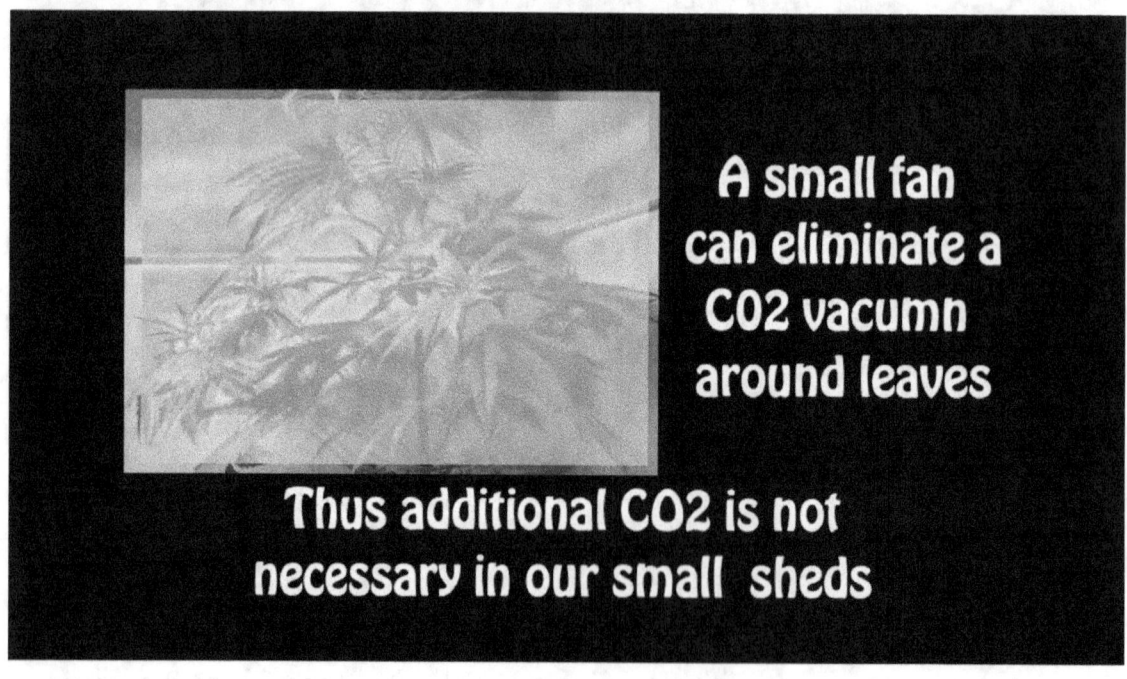

A small fan can eliminate a CO2 vacumn around leaves

Thus additional CO2 is not necessary in our small sheds

You may have heard that some growers add CO2 to their growing areas to promote growth. This might help a large garden but for a tiny medical marijuana garden we don't need it. If you have a fan as small as my Bahamas Breeze fan and it provides a steady stream of air around your plants they will have all the CO2 they will ever need. What does happen is that if you do not have a fan or some way to provide air movement around your plants the plant leaves can suck the CO2 out of the air and create a little CO2-less area around the leaves which can stop growth. The CO2 is the source of C (Carbon) which is the main building block of the plant. But a simple little fan along with the vent system we already installed will keep a constant supply of air and thus CO2 to our plants.

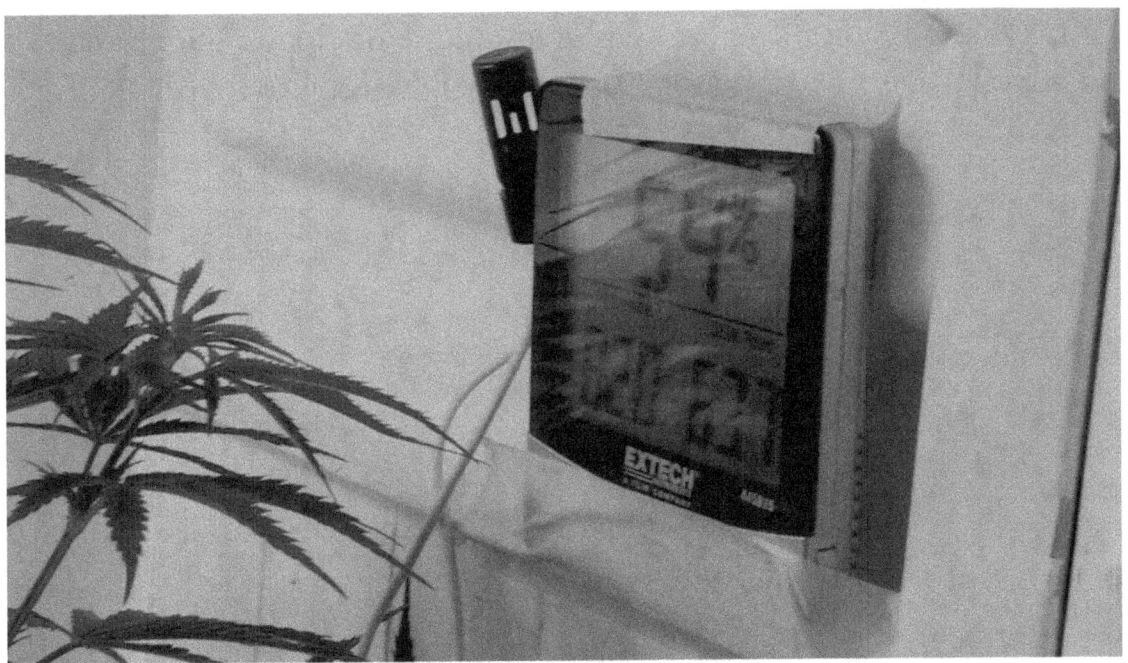

It is important to keep track of not only the humidity in our sheds but also the temperature. Here I have an Extech hygrometer taped to the wall of my bloom shed. Tape will keep the hygrometer from falling.

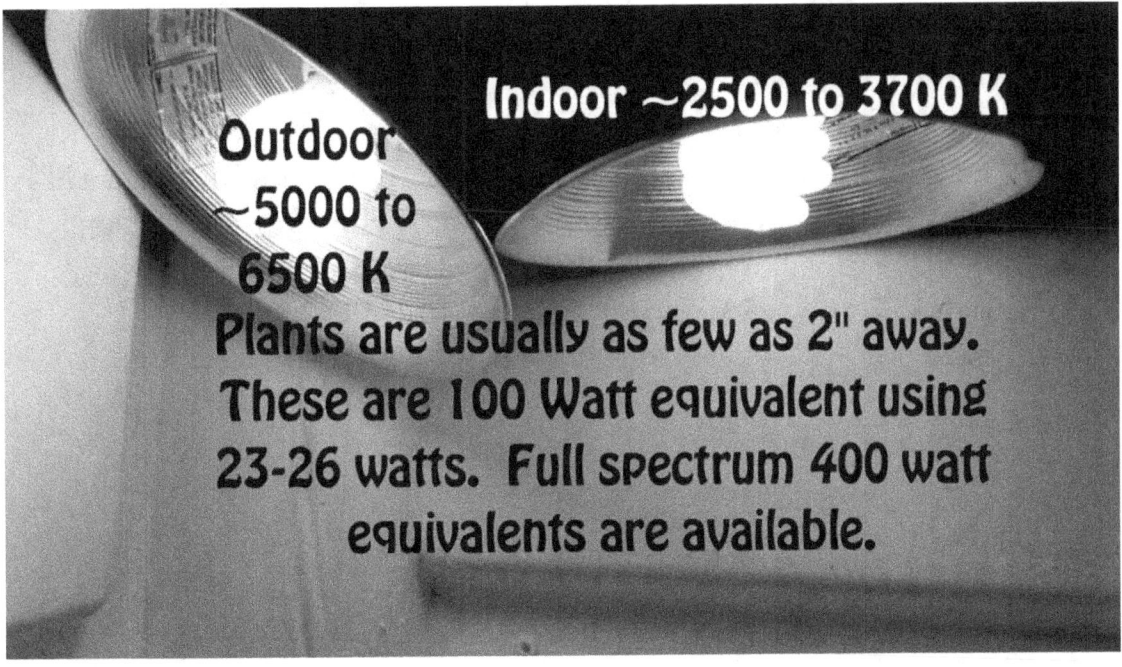

Indoor ~2500 to 3700 K

Outdoor ~5000 to 6500 K

Plants are usually as few as 2" away. These are 100 Watt equivalent using 23-26 watts. Full spectrum 400 watt equivalents are available.

I actually have a combination of lights that I use in my sheds. To start out two simple Compact Florescent Lights in my cans one around 6500 K and the other around 2700 K provide full spectrum. Depending on how hot they are you can get them very close to the plant. As close as

2" may be possible. The little CFLs are okay for clones and seedlings and even plants but for your bloom shed you'll want more light they can provide.

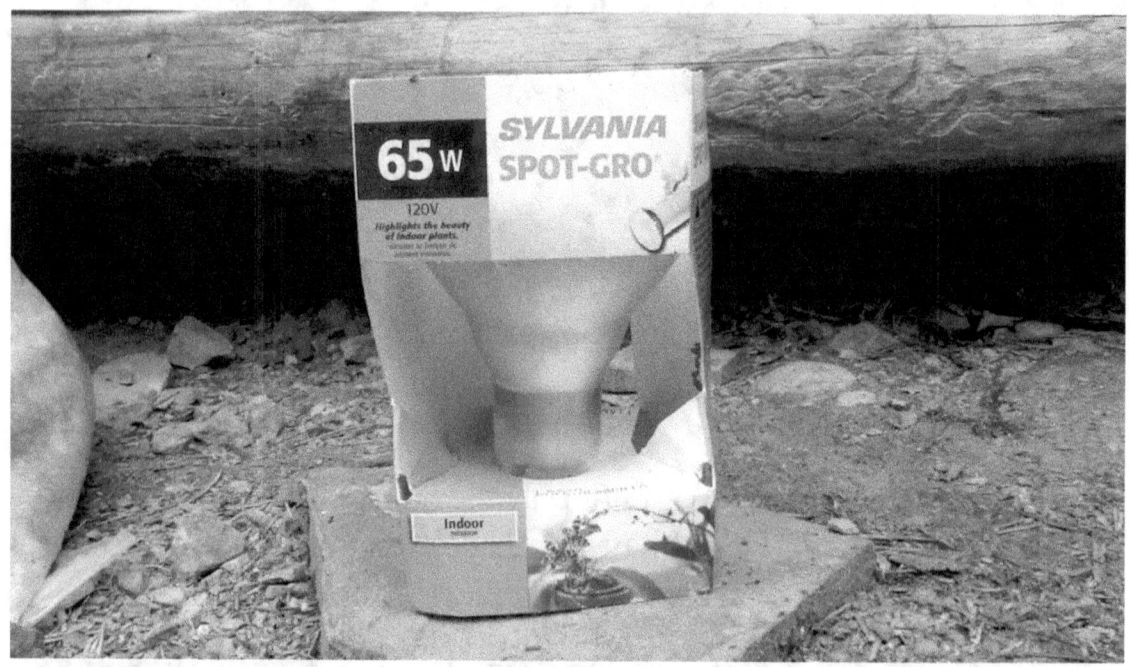

I added to Sylvania Spot-Gro's to my shed. This is a 65 watt full spectrum plant light. In theory this along with the CFLs could provide enough light for your shed. I actually use my spot-gro's for heat. But be careful with these. Keep them at least 12 inches from your plants. I killed at least one plant when a spot grow slipped. Make sure these spot gro's are secure and won't fall on your plants.

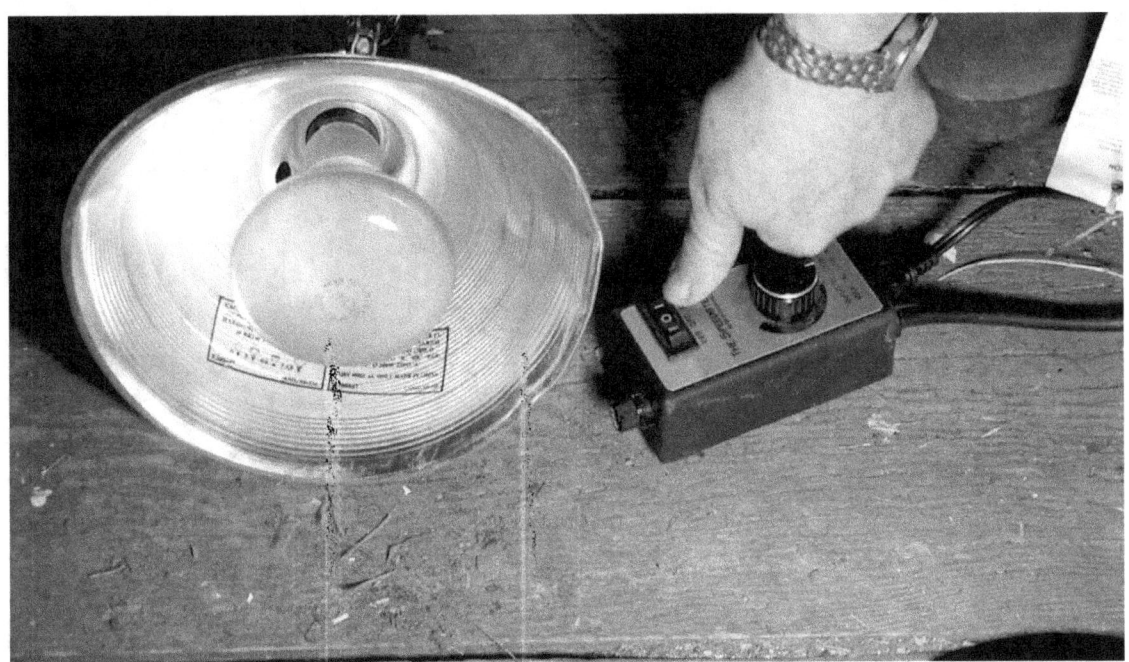

A power control may be usable with fans and lights, but make sure the lights and especially the fans can be used with them. For example, the power control works great with inline duct fans. But I found I did not need them for that. The little Bahamas Breeze fans WARN in the instructions not to use the fans with power controls to prevent risk of fire. Do READ the instructions on all of your equipment.

Above the control works great in controlling the heat put out by the spot-gro.

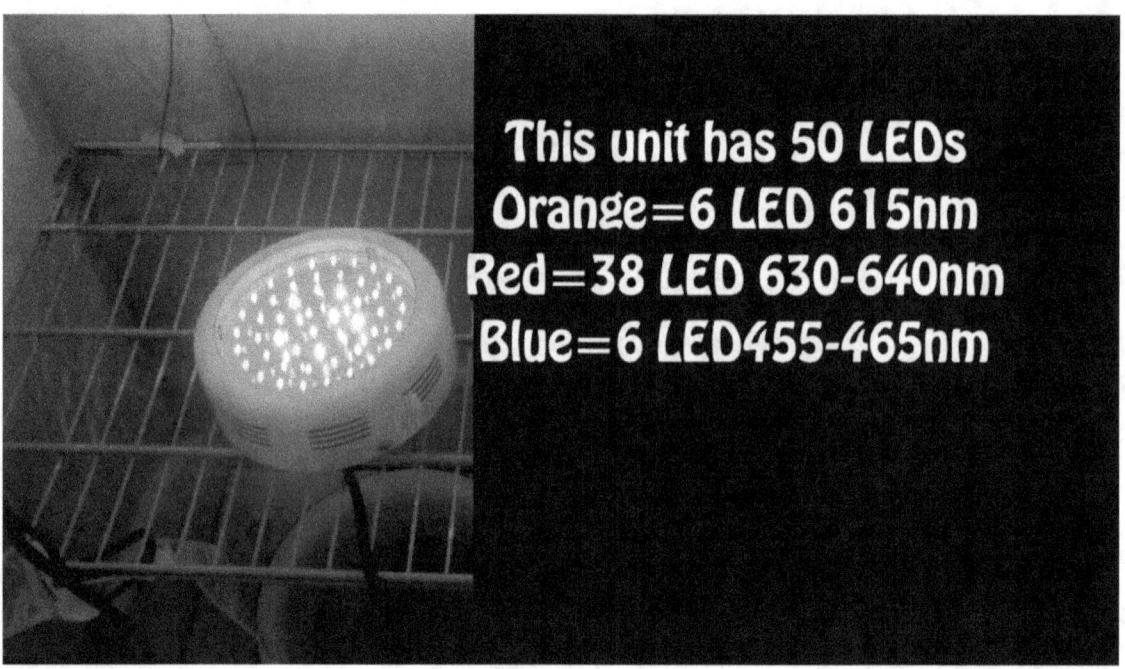

This unit has 50 LEDs
Orange=6 LED 615nm
Red=38 LED 630-640nm
Blue=6 LED455-465nm

But if you can afford it get yourself some LED lights. I started out with the 50 watt above and my plants loved it. Buy loving it I mean that the plants grew busy (lots of new branches and shoots) without getting very tall (Stretching happens when the plant has to look for more light.) We want to keep our plants as short as possible in the grow stage and the LED above is perfect for the grow shed.

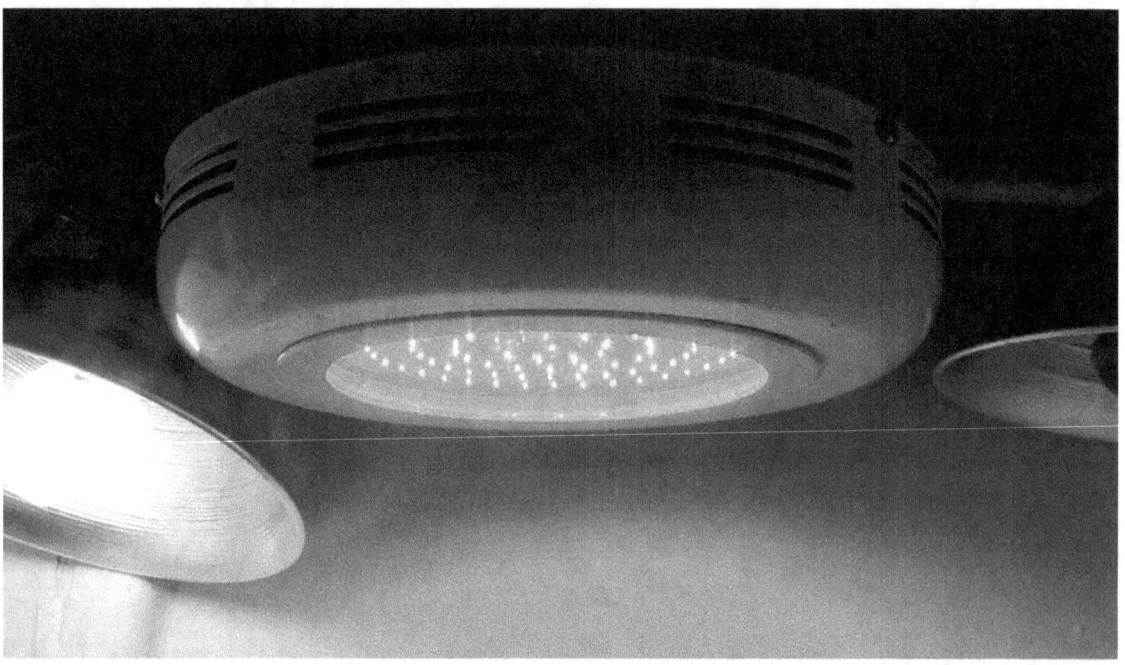

The 50 watt is perfect for my grow shed. However for our bloom shed I chose a 90 watt LED to provide even more light.

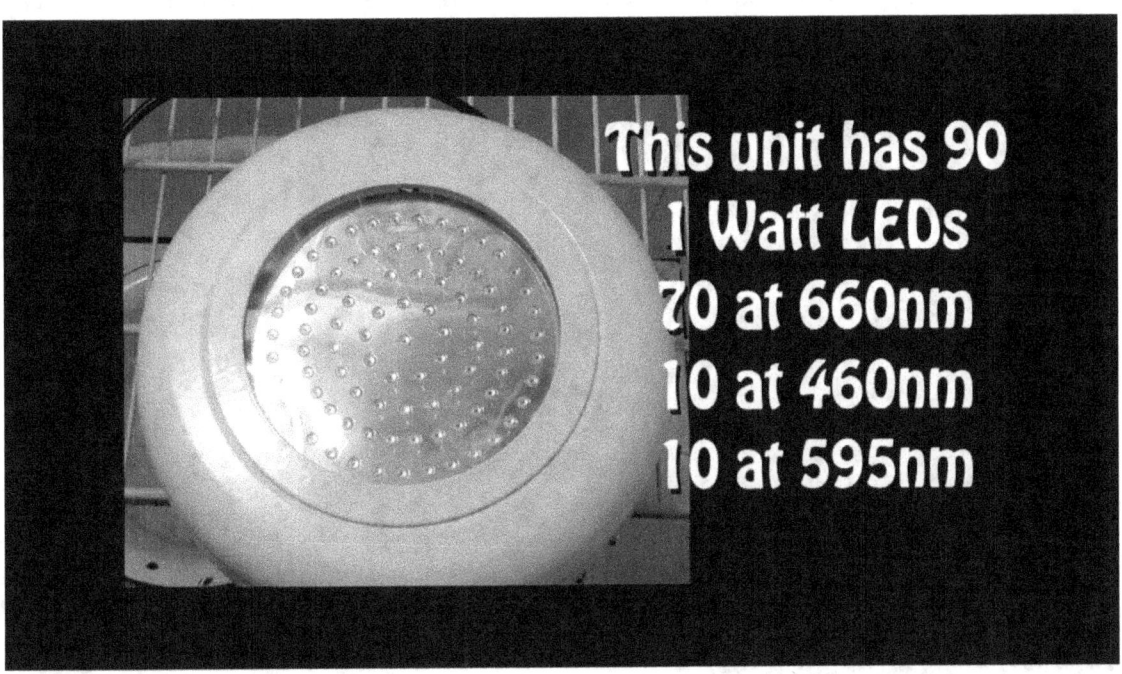

This 90 watt unit has 660 nm red rather than 630 nm red. The 660 is more suitable to blooming and the 630 more suitable for growing. Though a combination of both would work well in both bloom and grow sheds.

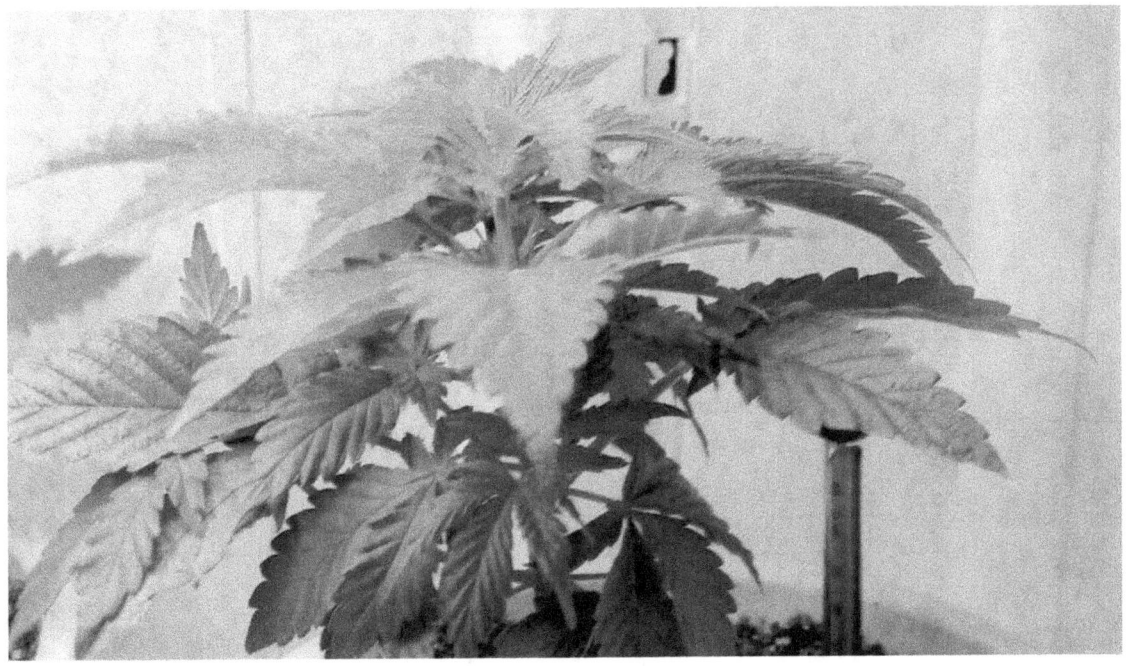

In this photo of a Church plant you can see that the plant has not grown high but there are many branches. This indicates the plant is getting the light it needs.

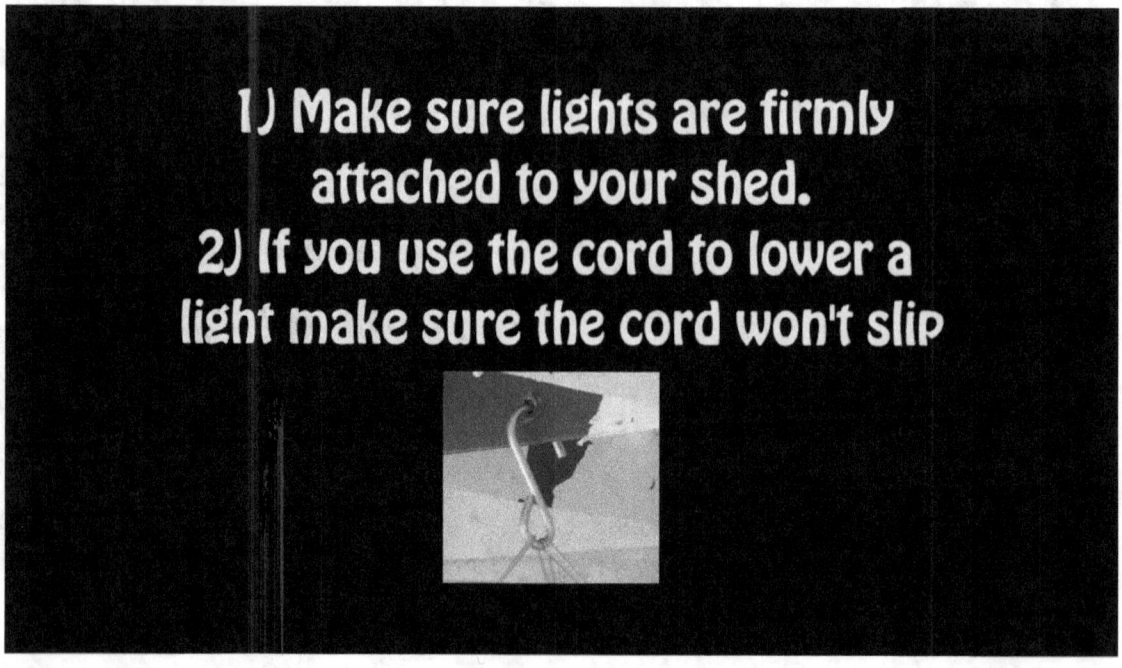

Do make sure all of your lights are firmly connected and won't slip. Hot lights falling can quickly kill a plant.

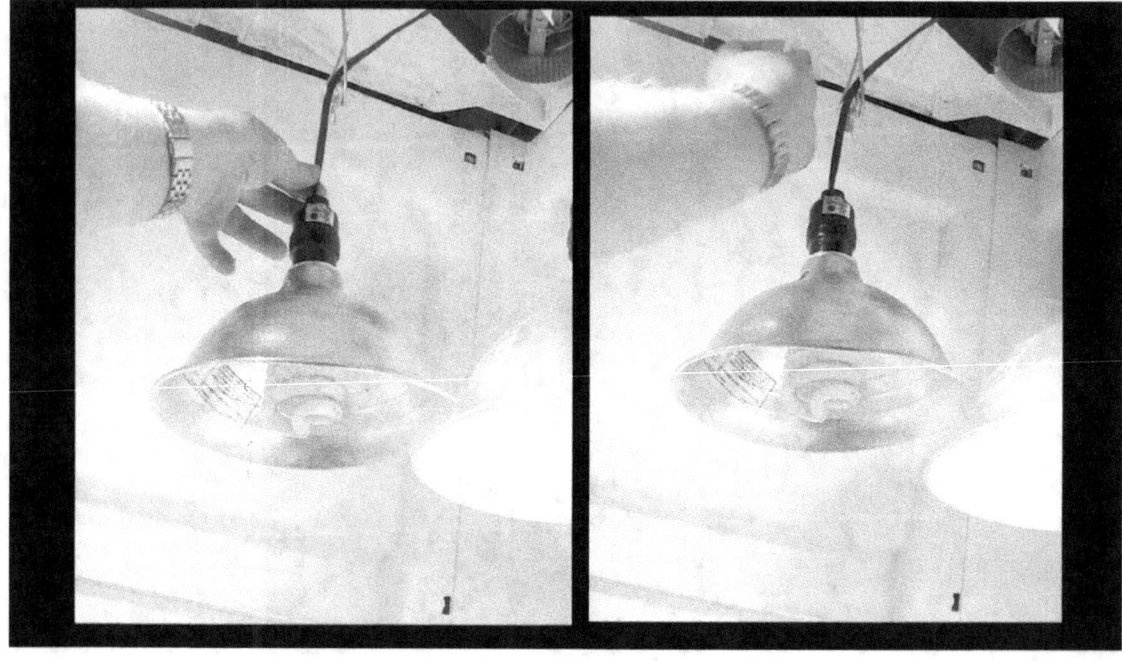

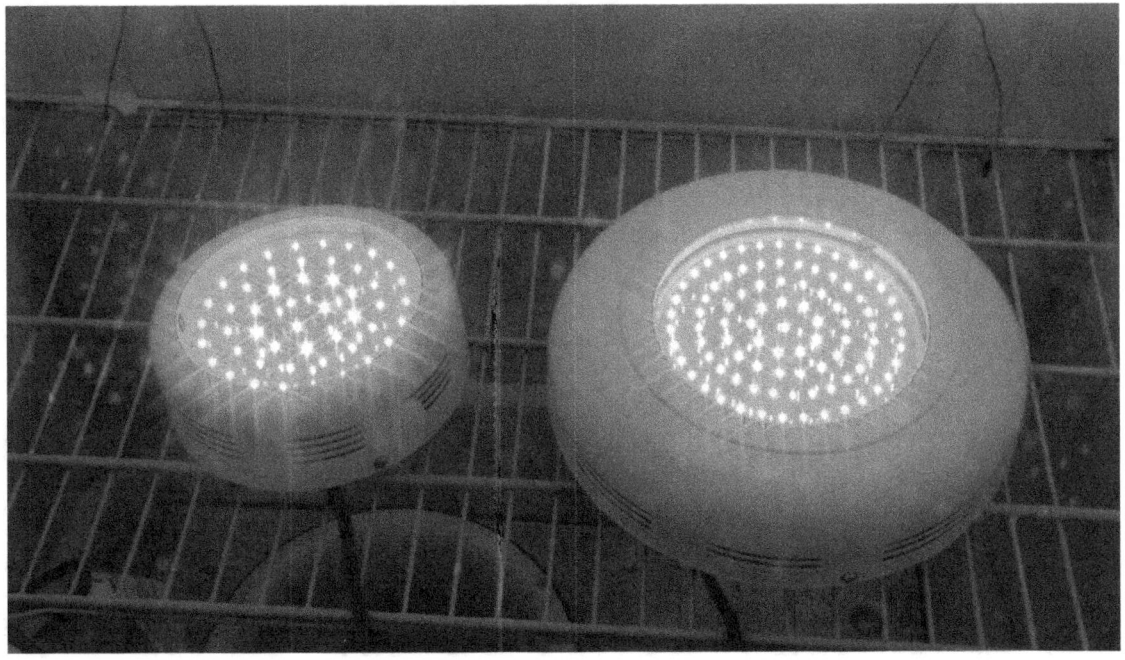

In the photo above you can see the size comparison of the 50 watt LED and the 90 watt LED.

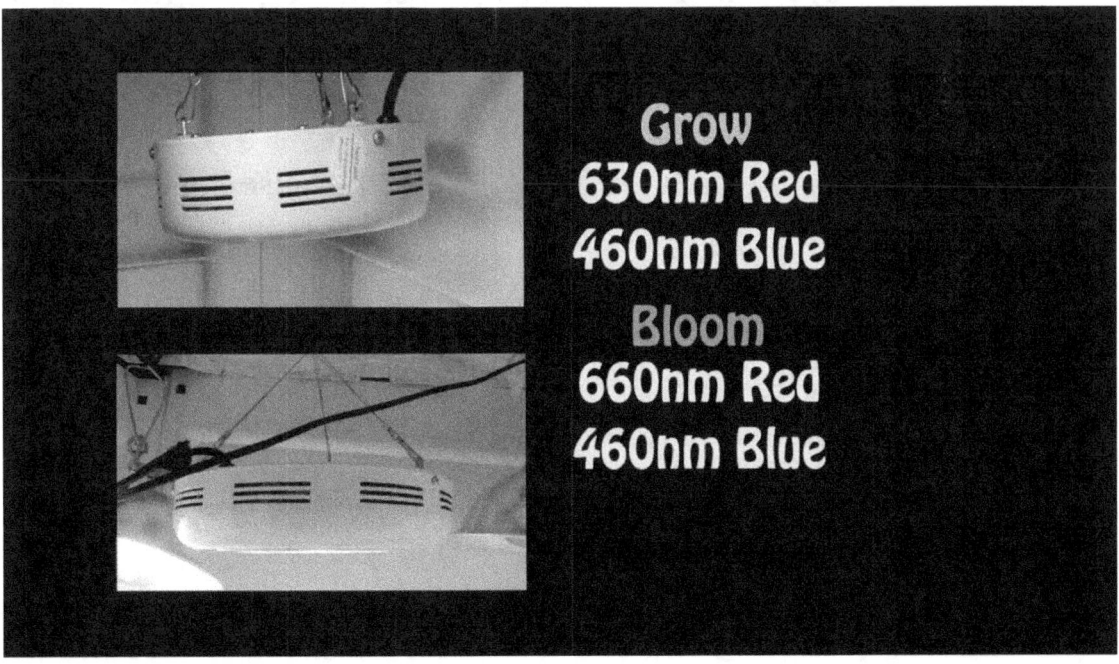

Grow
630nm Red
460nm Blue

Bloom
660nm Red
460nm Blue

The 50 watt is fine for my grow shed and the 90 watt is perfect for the bloom shed. LED lights can get very close to the plants and they usually have built in fans and never get very hot.

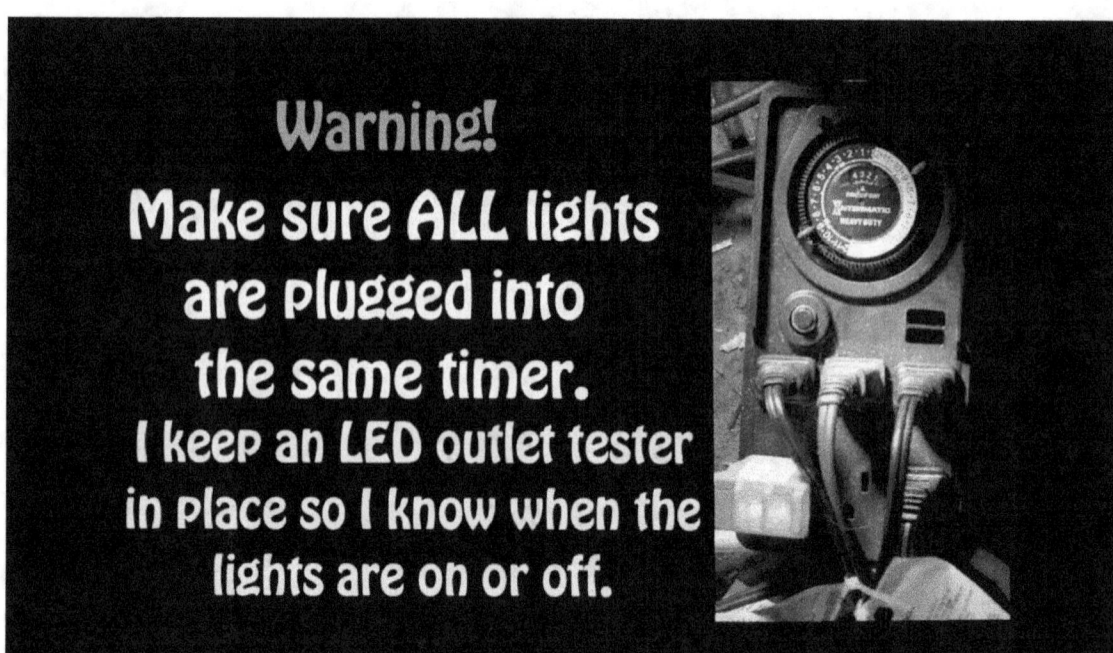

Warning!

Make sure ALL lights are plugged into the same timer.

I keep an LED outlet tester in place so I know when the lights are on or off.

No matter what lights you use make sure all the lights for one shed are plugged into the same timer. I use both digital and pin timers (a pin timer is shown above) and find the pin timers easier to set. However, a bump to the timer can cause the time to bump—i.e. you set a timer from 9 to 9 for the bloom shed. You bump it accidentally. Now the timer comes on at 9:20 AM and goes off at 9:20 PM. It still measures out 12 hours but the start and stop times have changed because the timer was bumped.

WARNING: Be sure to check your timers if you have any power outages that might affect your times.

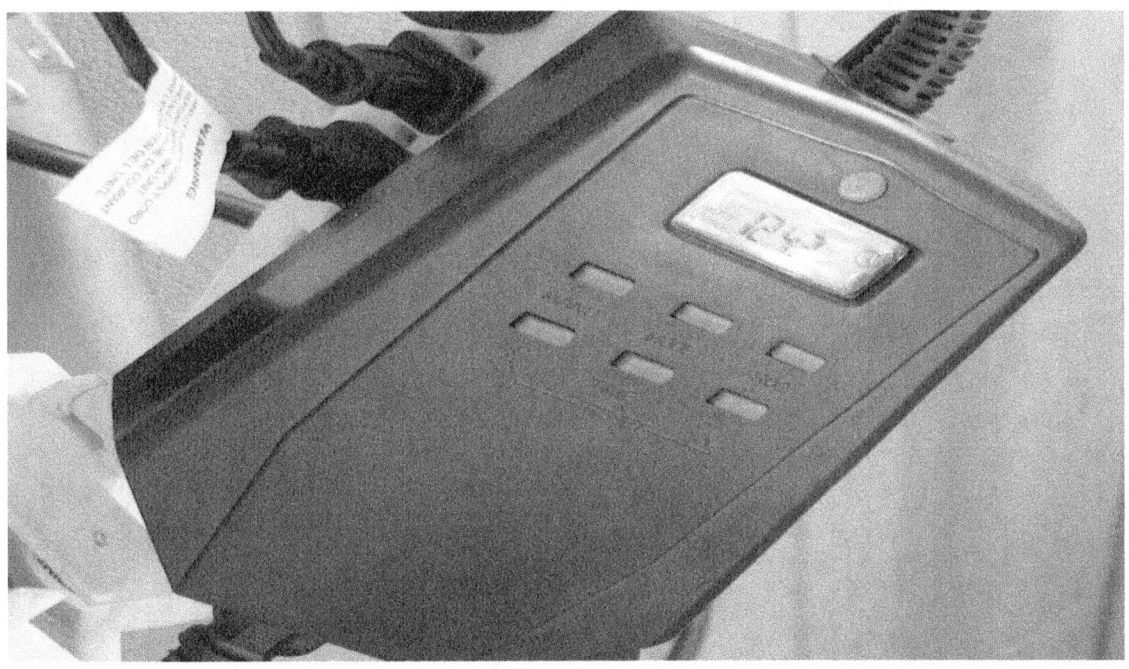

Digital timers also work well. They also need to be checked if there are any power outages.

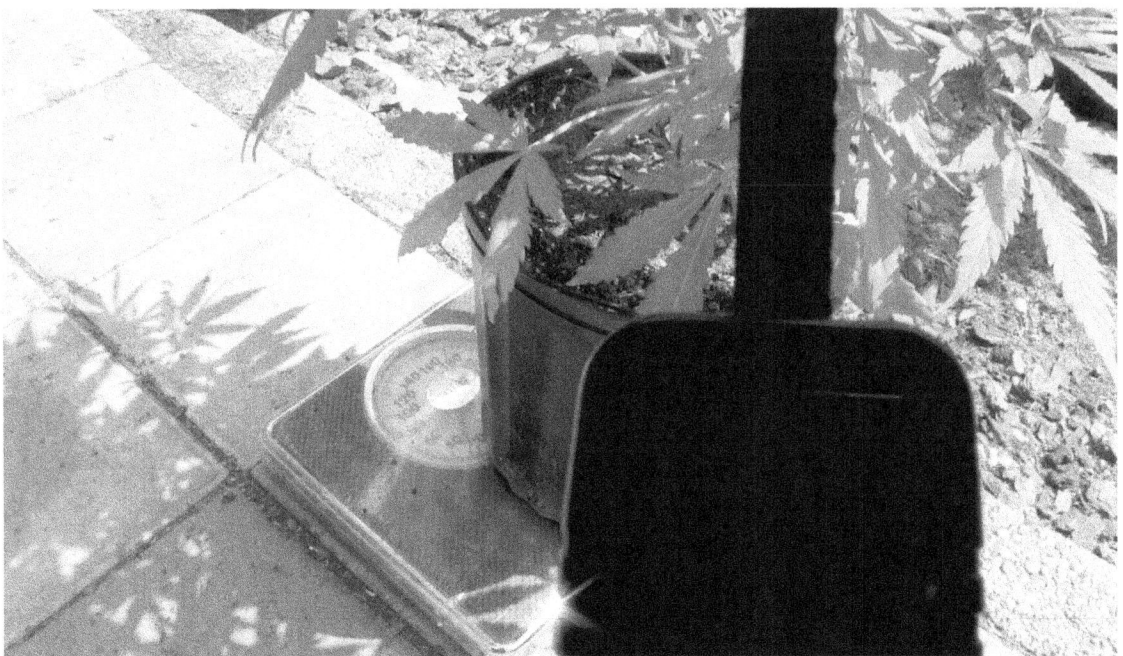

When building your sheds keep in mind that marijuana plants, especially in big pots can weight many pounds. Be sure that your shelves, etc, in your grow shed can take the weight of multiple pots.

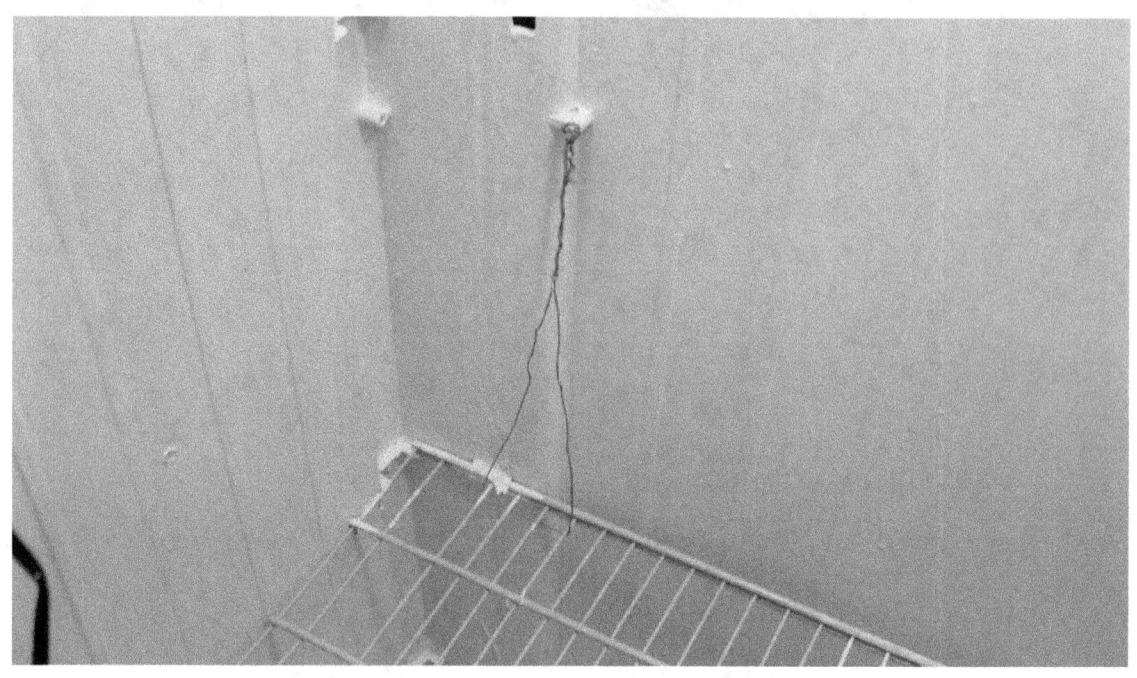

I used wire and even wooden braces to make sure my shelves didn't fall. A tipped over pot will spill your dirt and may harm your plant. So make sure your shed can take the weight of your pots.

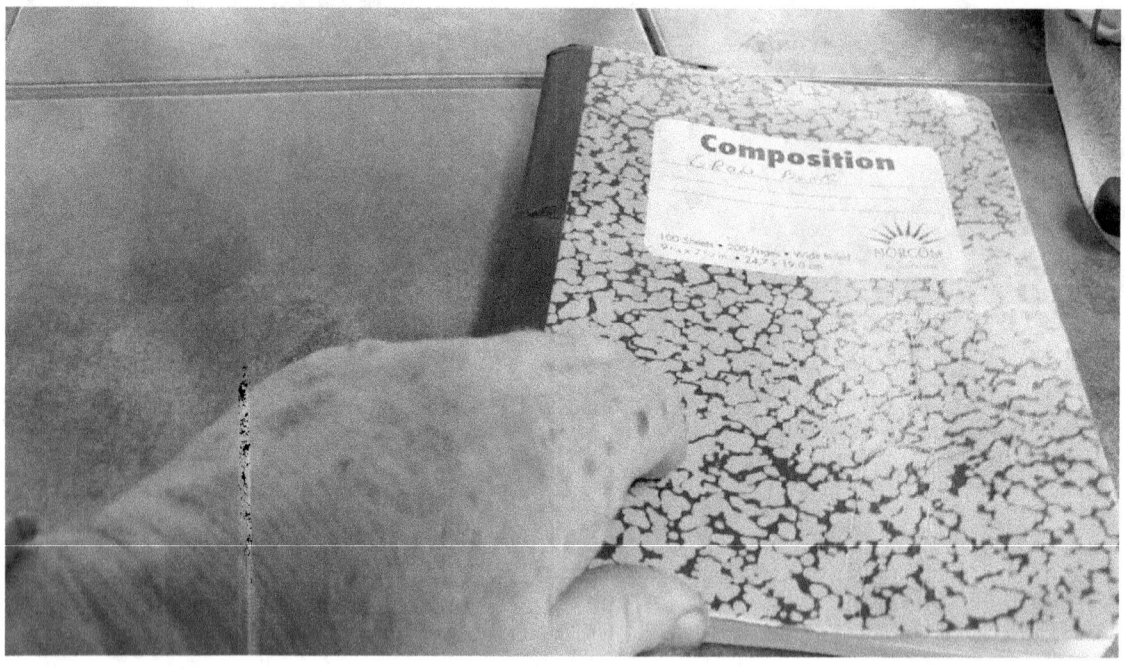

Do yourself a favor and keep a grow diary. In it write down: the soil mix you use,the fertilizer you use; the temperature and humidity in your grow and bloom cabinets during the day. (You'll need to write down temperature and humidity more often in the beginning. As you become more experienced in regulating the temperature and humidity of your sheds you won't need to check as often.) And anything else you can think of. I keep formulas for my fertilizer mix on the last page so I don't have to repeat writing them down.

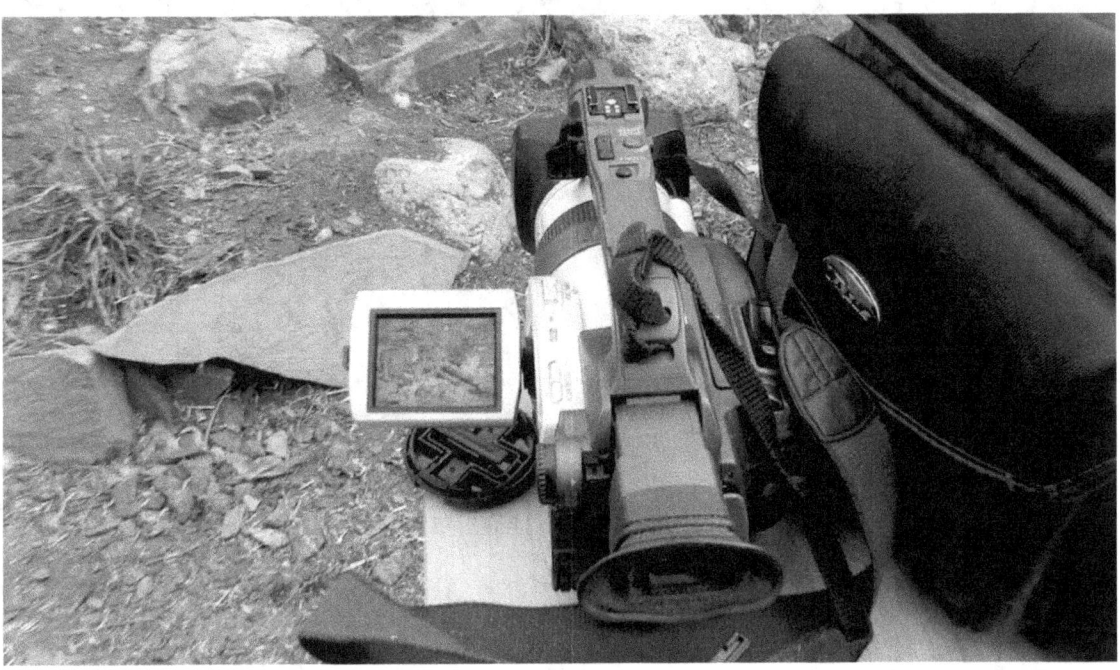

If you have any kind of digital camera take photos of your plants every day. This will come in handy when you begin to wonder how a previous clone was doing, say 20 days after it came out of the humidity dome, or how large a different seedling had grown.

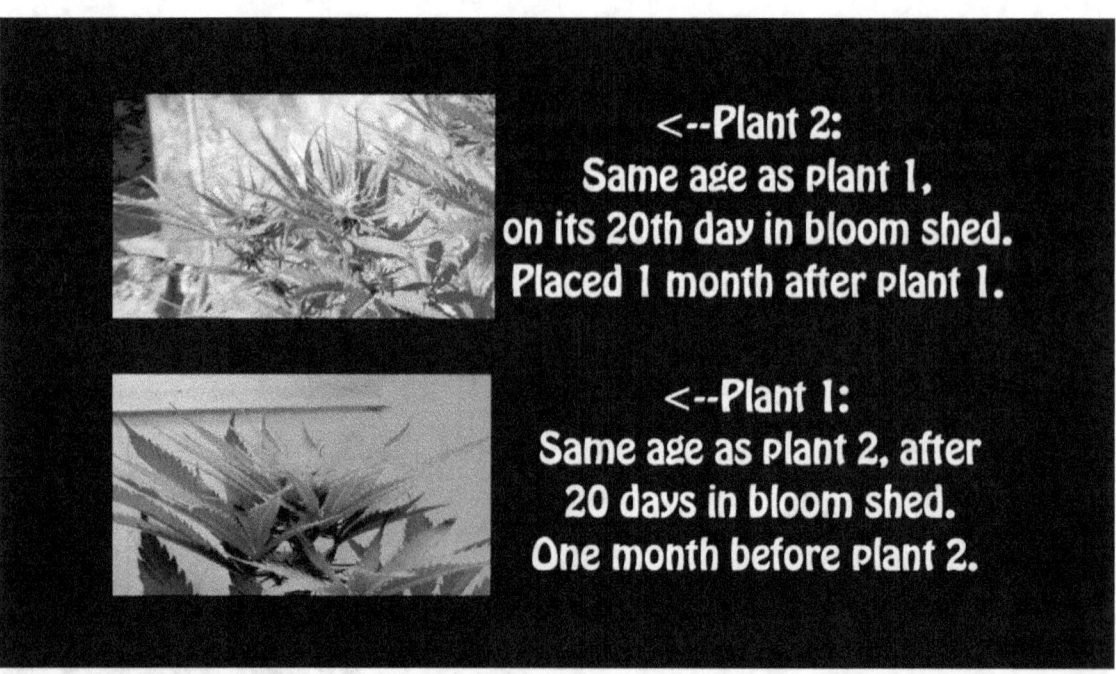

<--Plant 2:
Same age as plant 1,
on its 20th day in bloom shed.
Placed 1 month after plant 1.

<--Plant 1:
Same age as plant 2, after
20 days in bloom shed.
One month before plant 2.

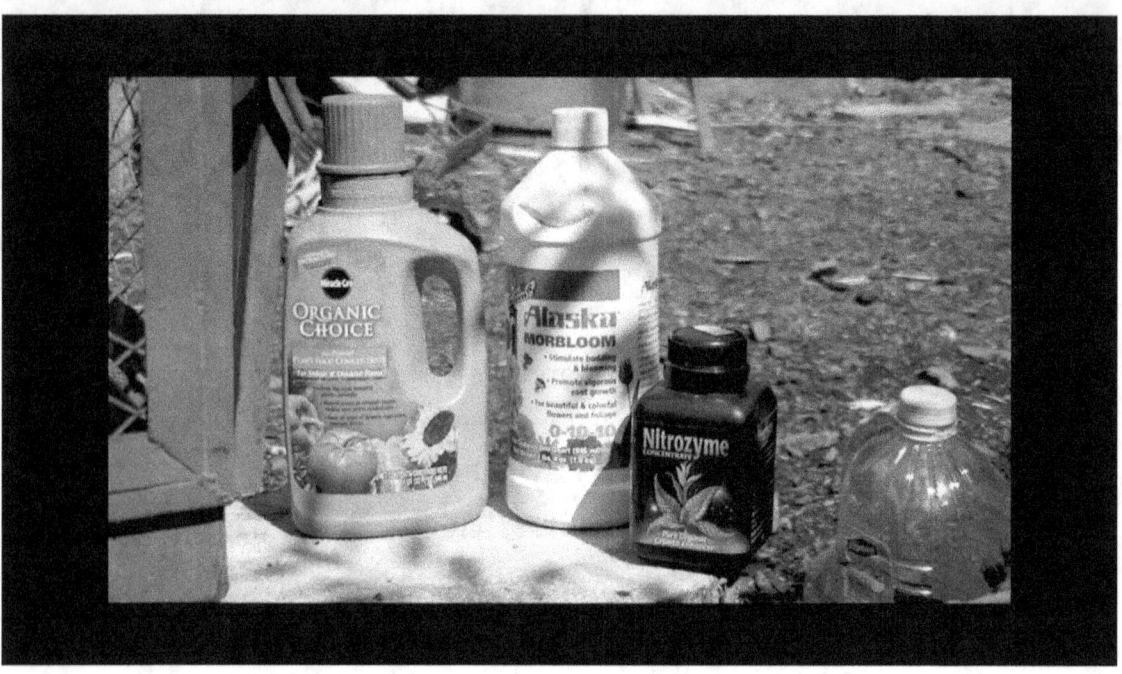

For my fertilizers I wanted something I could get at any hardware store.
And for the most part that worked out. I choose Miracle Grow
Organic Choice as my main growing fertilizer and Alaska Morbloom 0-
10-10 for my bloom shed fertilizer.   To enhance growth I used
Nitrosyme a seaweed extract sold in the UK. Sources for Nitrosyme
can be found on my website. http://learntogrowmedicalmarijuana.com.

Liquid Seaweed is a good substitute for Nitrosyme that you might find in a local garden centers.

The Nitrosyme which I used to soak seed, soak my soilless mix, and as a foliar fertilizer enhances growth and actually took one entire week off the growing time of my marijuana.

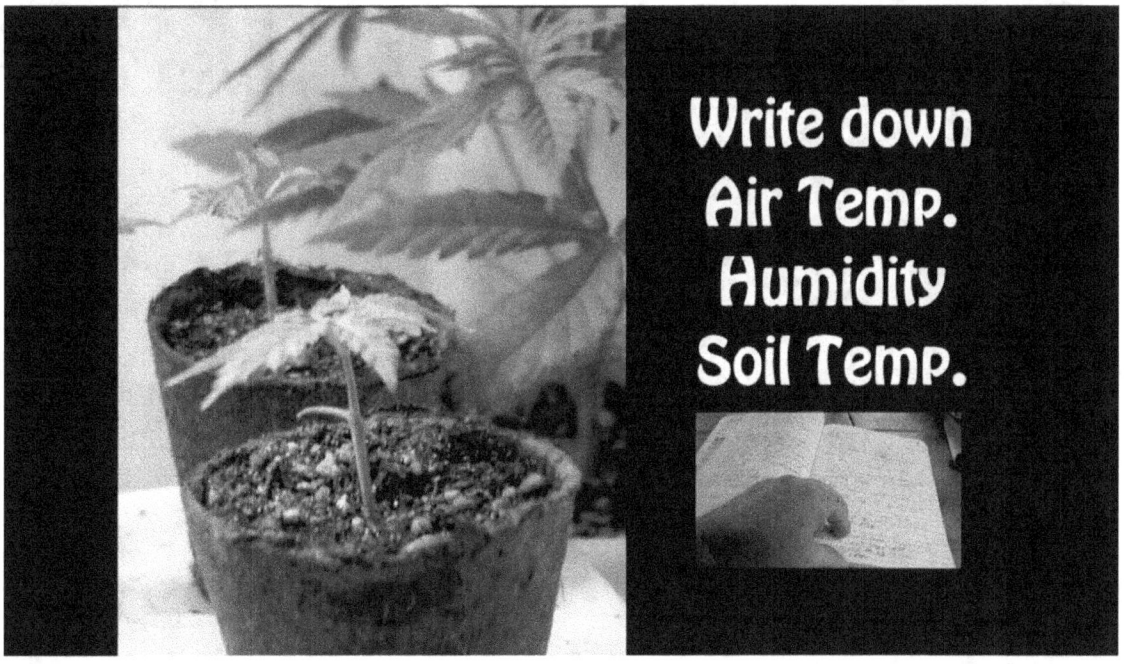

You can learn a great deal more by writing your experiences down and using them as a learning tool.

My first marijuana plants did not survive.

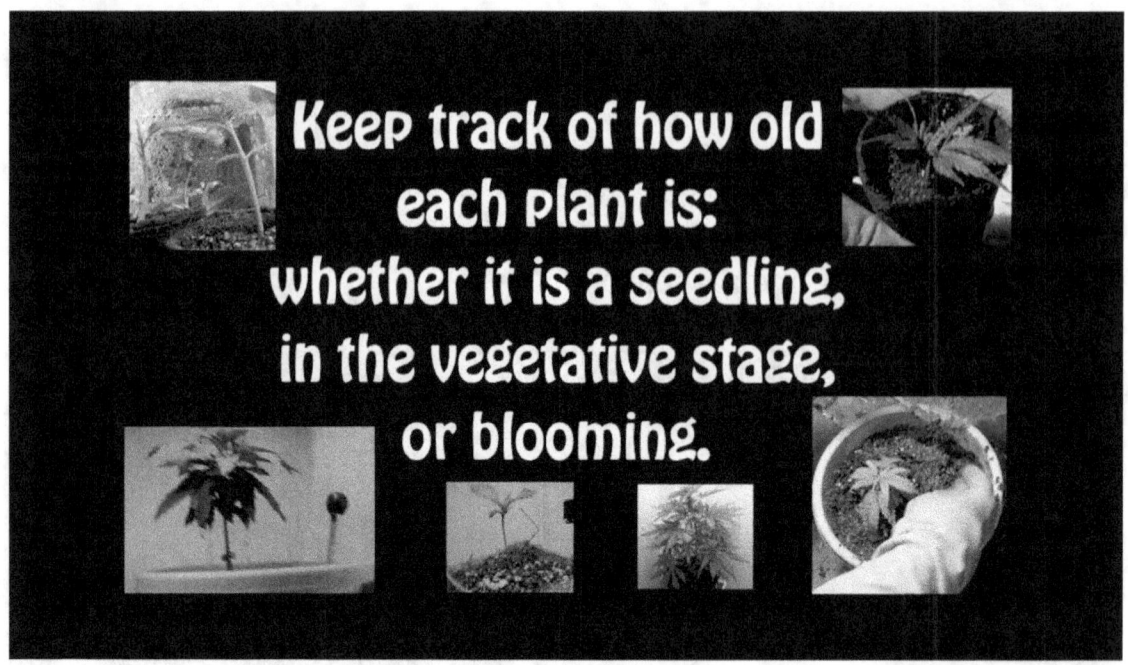

Keep track of how old
each plant is:
whether it is a seedling,
in the vegetative stage,
or blooming.

Do, of course, figure out a system of keeping track of each plants. Name them, number them. Just always make it clear which plant is which. Keeping track of how long a plant has been in the bloom shed will give you a good idea when to stop fertilizing (many grower's use only water for the last ten days of blooming to reduce fertilizer taste.)

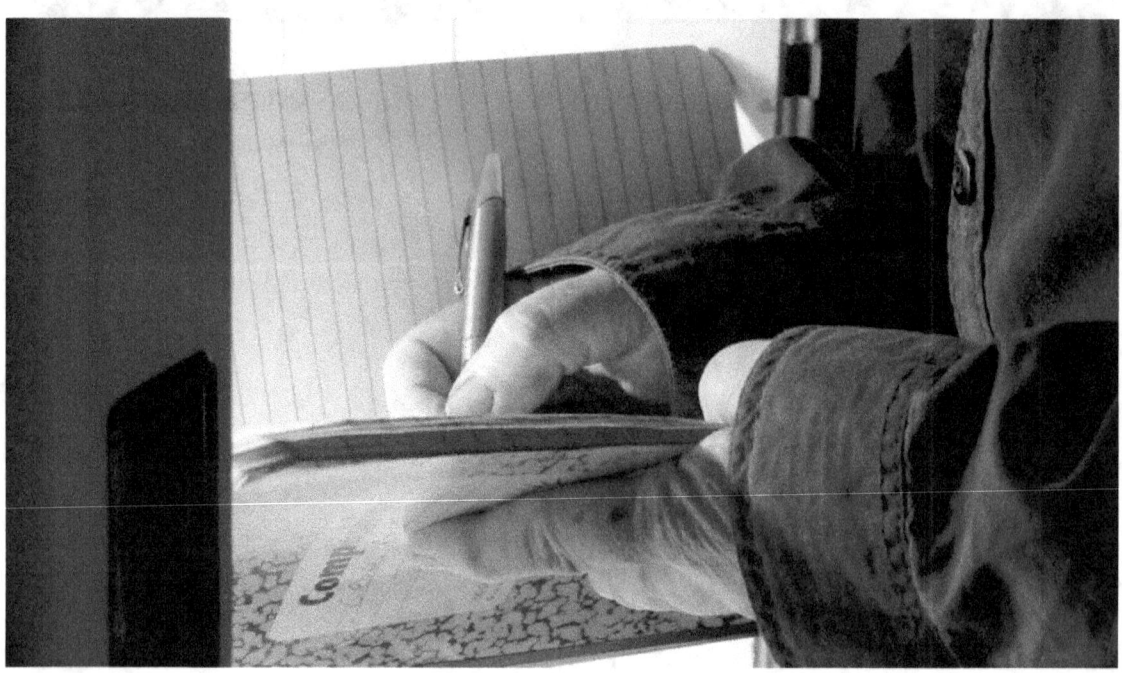

If you keep the notebook by your sheds and make a habit of writing things down, your notebook will provide you with a wealth of knowledge for future growing.

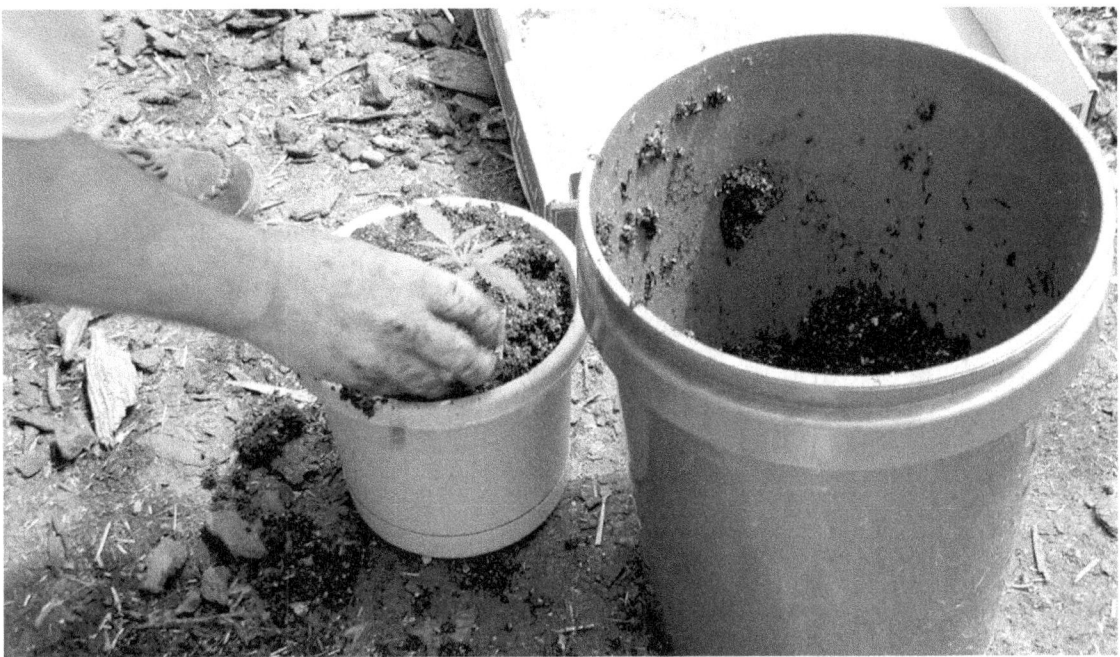

For my plants I choose a soil-less mix. Soil-less meaning a soil which does not have any nutrient content for the plants. This allows us to control the nutrients and control plant growth.

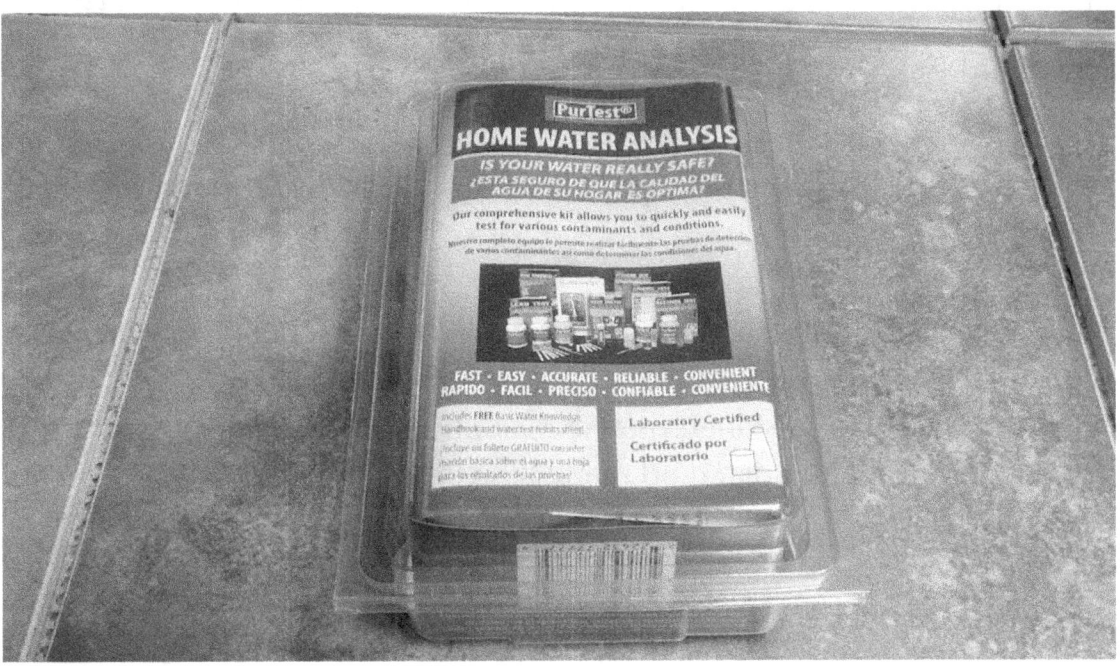

The first thing you need to do is check your water. With a soil-less system hard water will not be as much of a problem as it would be in say a hydroponics system. In fact, one of the reasons for choosing soil-less is that it has many of the benefits of hydroponics without the disadvantages. That is we can control our nutrients, but an error will not be fatal to all of our plants.

One thing you do have to look out for as far as water is concerned is chlorine. Sometimes added to city water to purify it, chlorine can inhibit growth. If you do find you have chlorine in your water you will need to do something about removing it or find another water source.

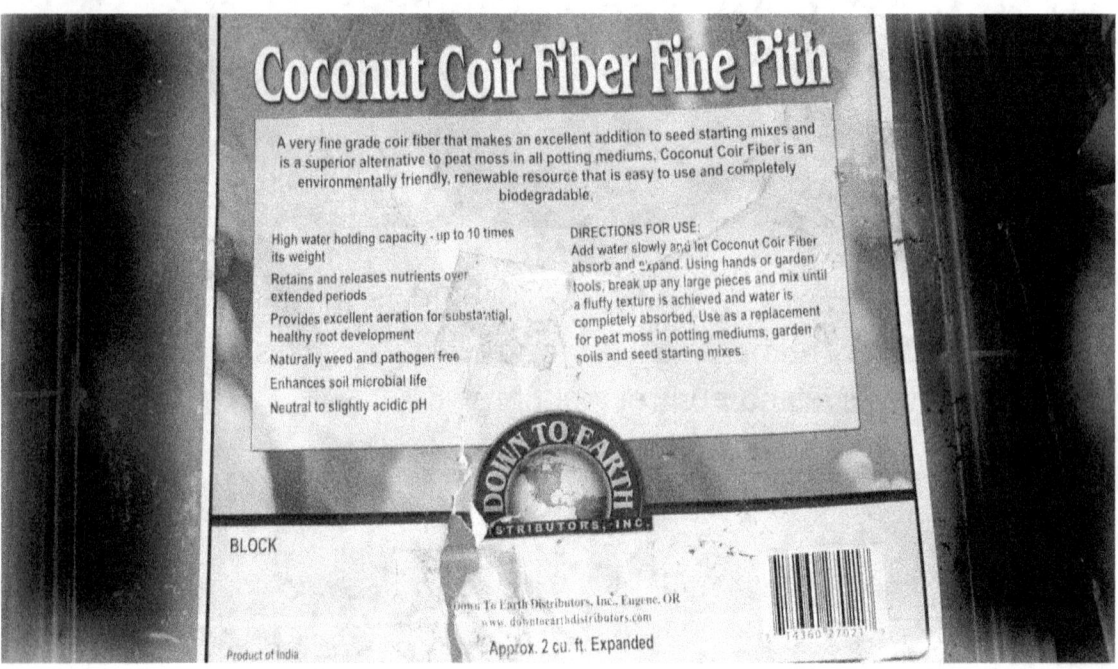

My soil-less mix consists of five ingredients used in equal measure, chosen because they are fast draining, but also because they hold moisture well. The first ingredient is Coconut Coir. This is fiber from the coconut plant and can hold many times its weight in water.

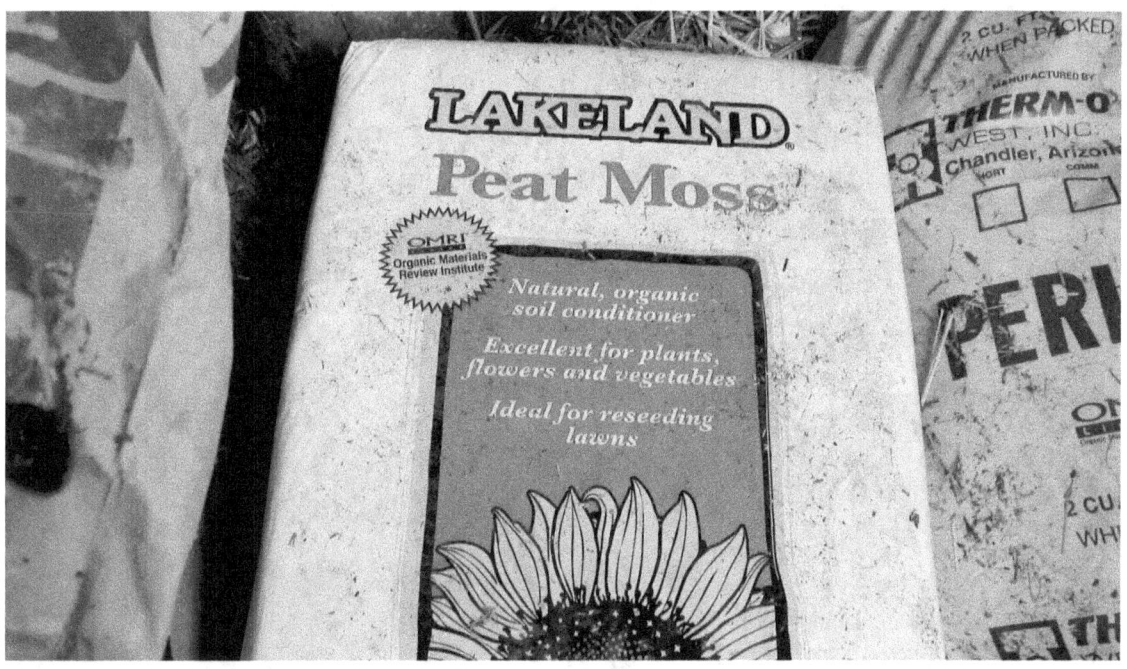

Similar to the Coir is my next ingredient Peat Moss. In fact it you could use two parts Coir or two parts Peat Moss instead of one serving of each. However, because I used coir and peat pots and like my roots to find something they are familiar with on the other side of their original container when they grow out, I use a coir/peat mix.

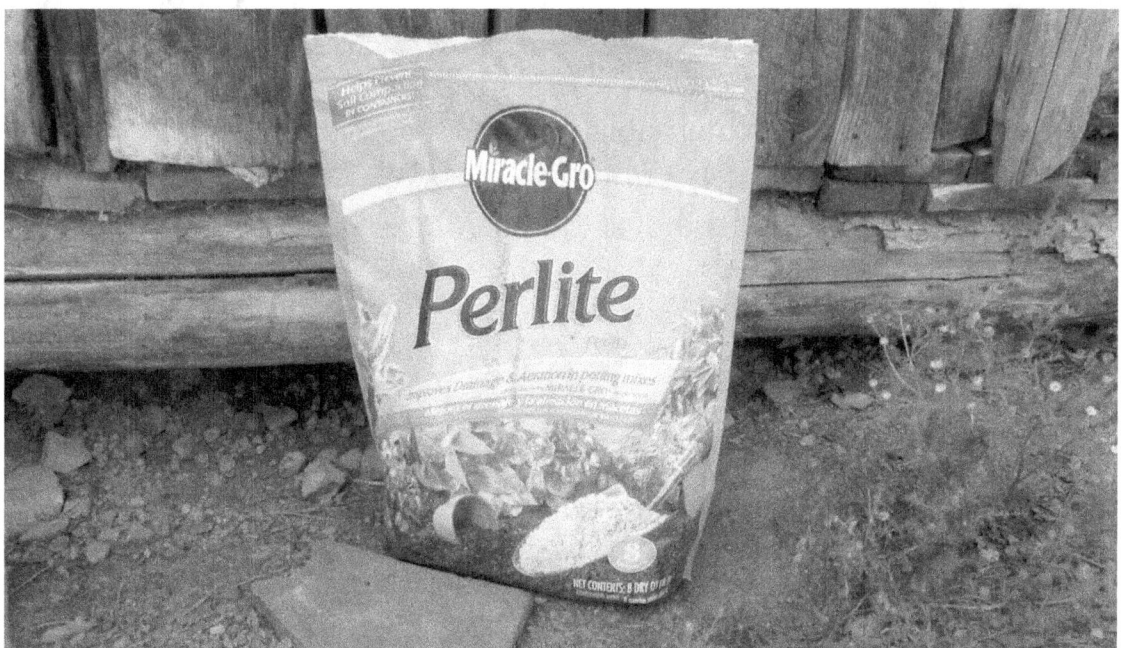

The next ingredient is Perlite. Perlite contributes to how well the soil drains and the little facets in the perlite pieces trap oxygen which plant roots need to grow. Do check the Perlite you buy. The original Perlite I purchased contained chemicals which gave off ammonia. Ammonia raises pH and I had to add Natural (pH) Up in order to keep my pH in the 6.0 range that is best for marijuana growing.

When making a mix for seedlings I crush large Perlite pieces so that they don't overwhelm the seedlings.

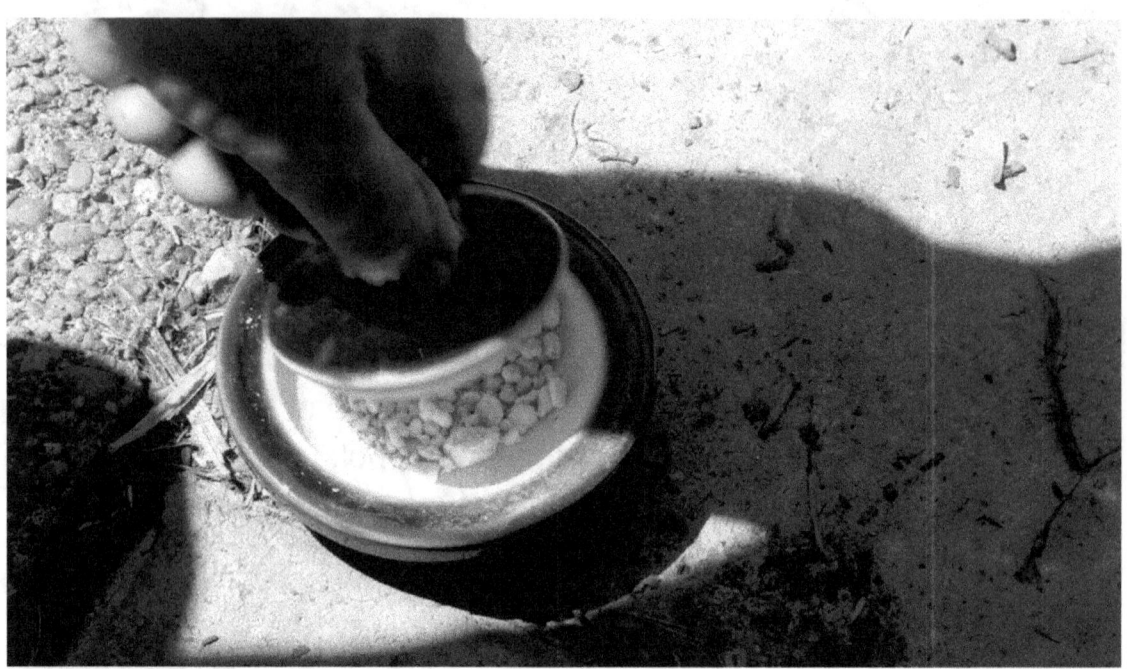

Sand contributes to the drain-ability of our soil. And also gives the soil a very unique dry feel when it does dry out. With experience you can check your soil moisture with just a touch of a finger.

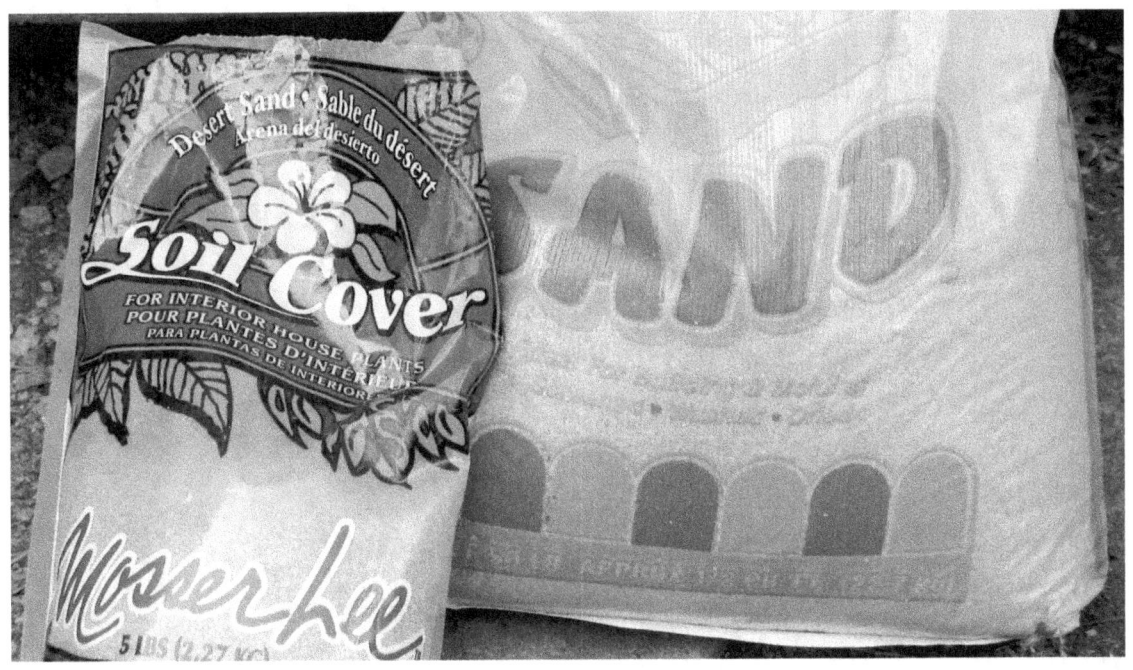

Make sure you sand it desert sand. Beach sand contains salt and that is not good for planting.

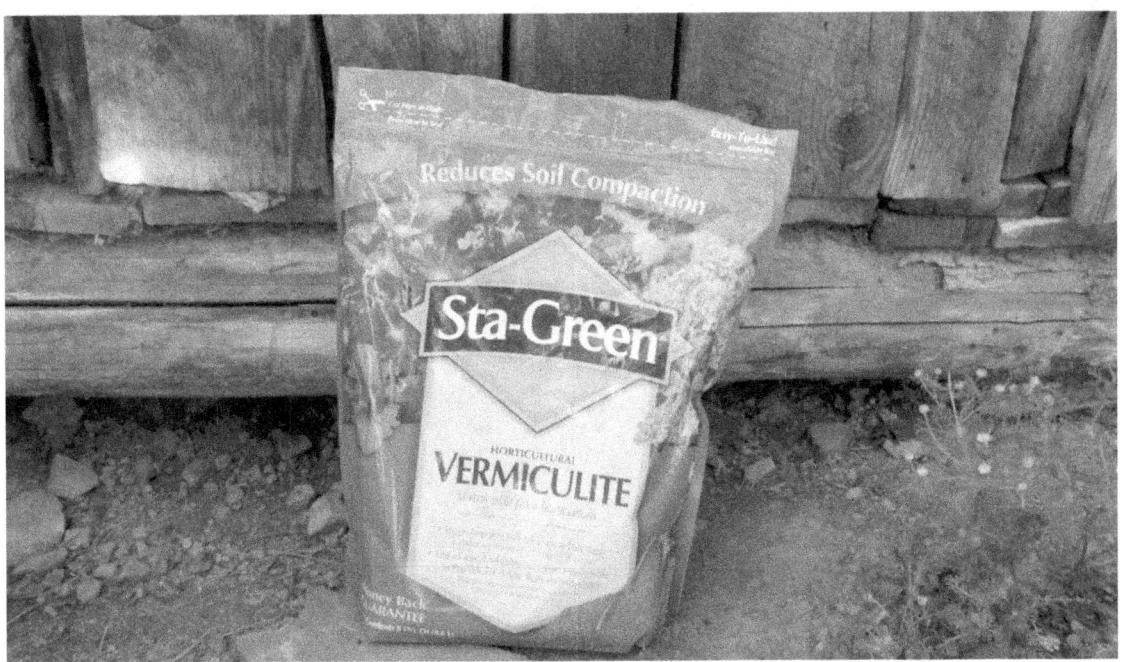

My next ingredient is Vermiculite. This material holds many times its weight in water and helps provide needed moisture.

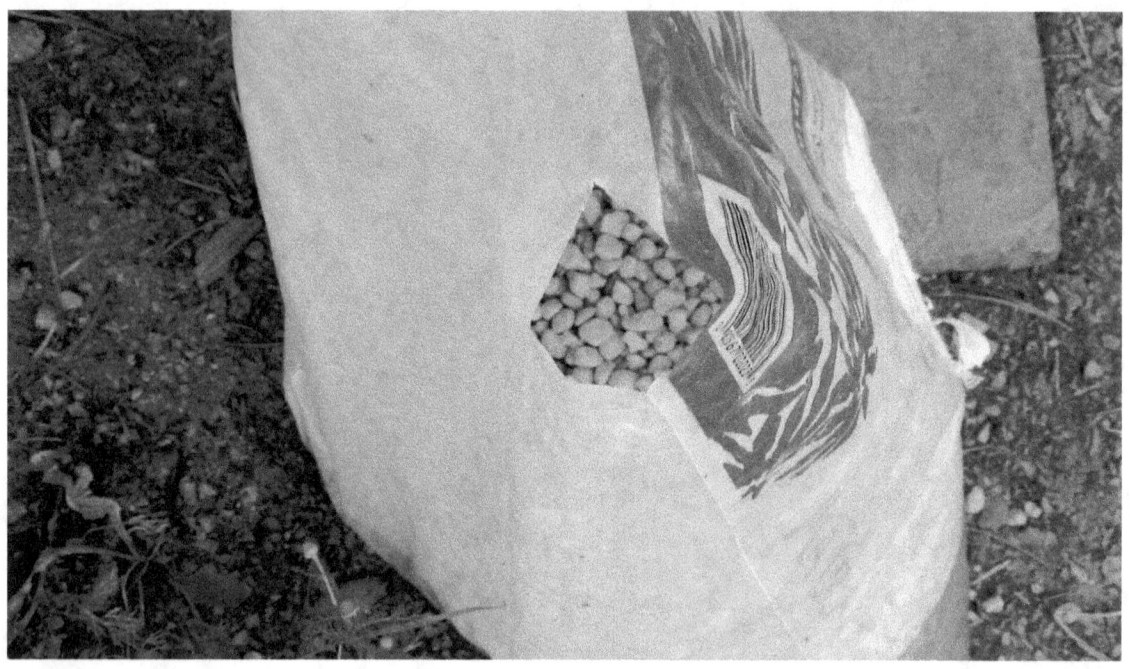

Don't forget pebbles for the bottom of your pot. This helps with drainage.

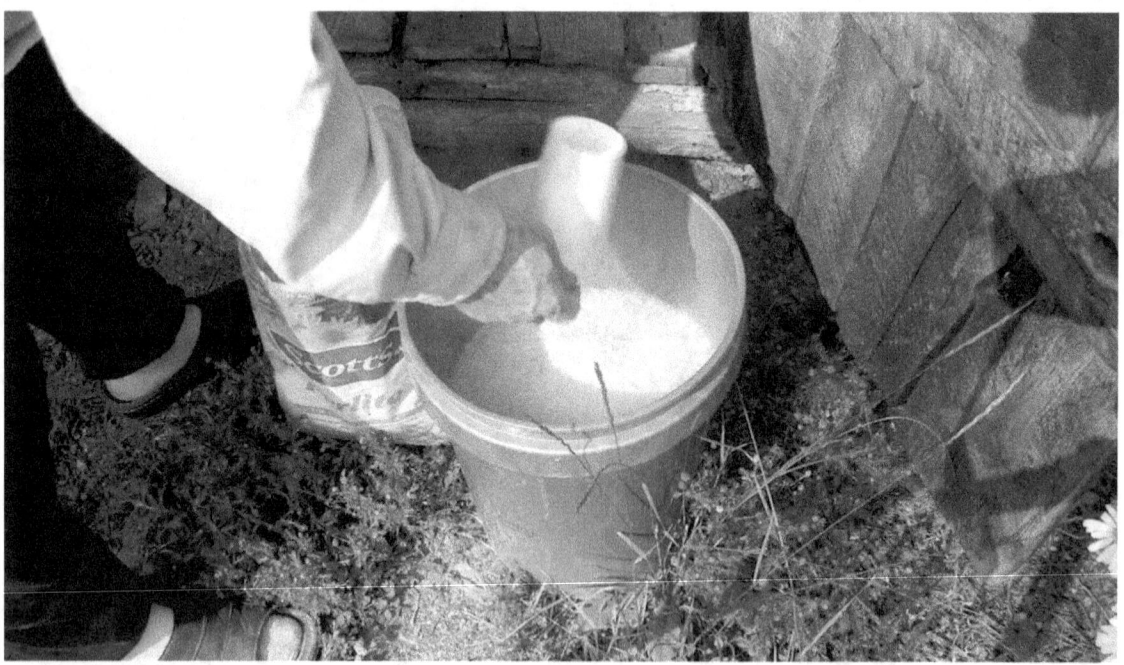

I mix equal portions of my five dry ingredients in a 5 gallon bucket. Adding plenty of water to make sure that the Coir, Peat and Vermiculite have the opportunity to absorb all the water they possibly can.

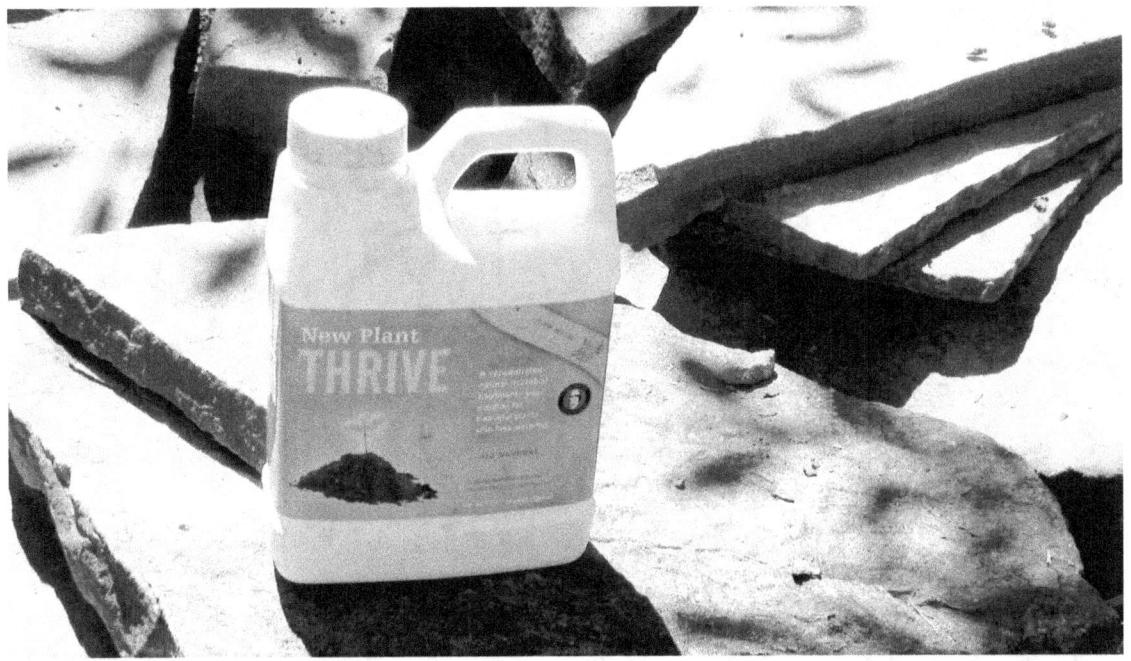

My background was writing about ginseng farming and with ginseng it was necessary to fumigate the soil after a crop if you wanted to plant again in the same garden. When you fumigate you take out all organisms. Nature abores a vacumn and if you eliminate all soil organisms new ones can move in, and sometimes those new organisms will be bad ones.

Our soil-less mix does not contain soil organisms and to make it harder for bad soil organisms to thrive I add THRIVE. This is a mixture of bacteria and fungi that make a soil-less mix more like real soil to the advantage of our plants.

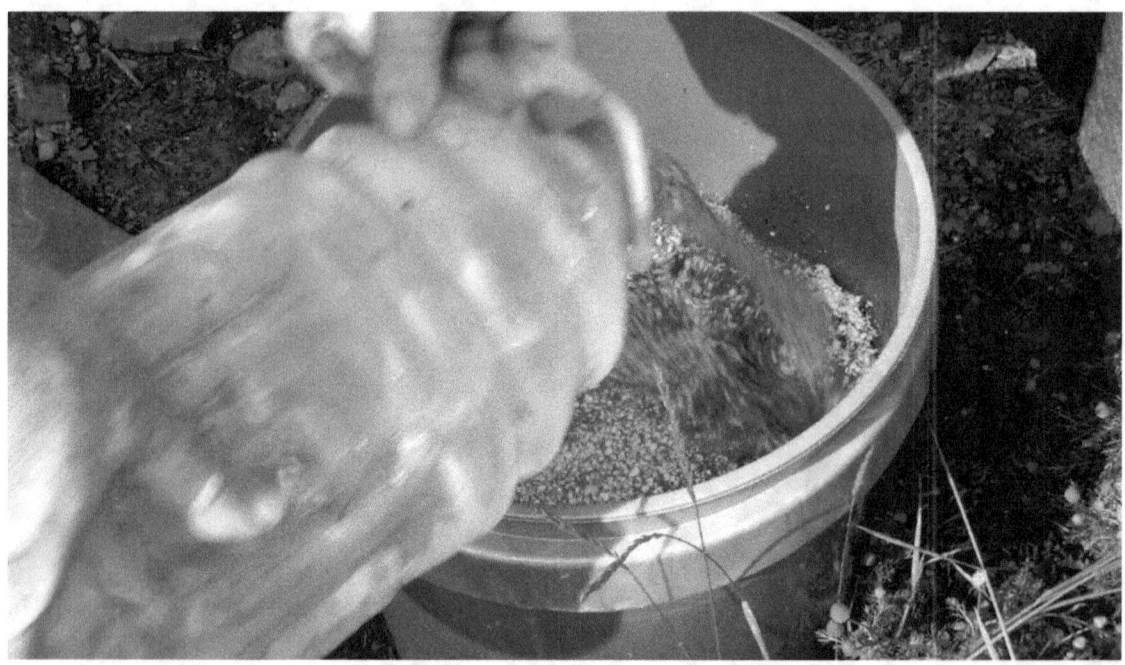

I mix my water in and stir by hand, adding the thrive after the water has been added.

H ion concentration
Medical Marijuana pH Range
7.5 on the high side
6.0 on the low side
5.5-6.0 for clones
pH can affect marijuana growth!

I also check the pH of the soil. The pH is the hydrogen ion concentration and indicates the acidity of our soil-less mix. When first mixed our ingredients should be around pH 7.

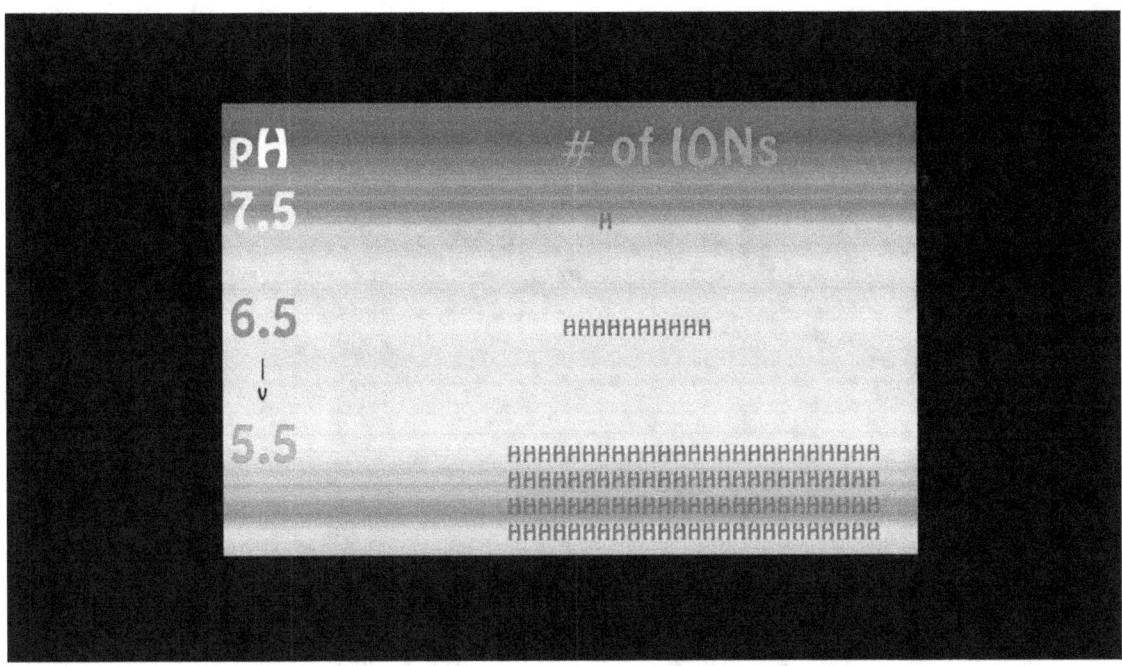

However, if your Perlite contains Ammonia the pH will be higher. What we want is a pH of about 6.0 for the best marijuana growth.

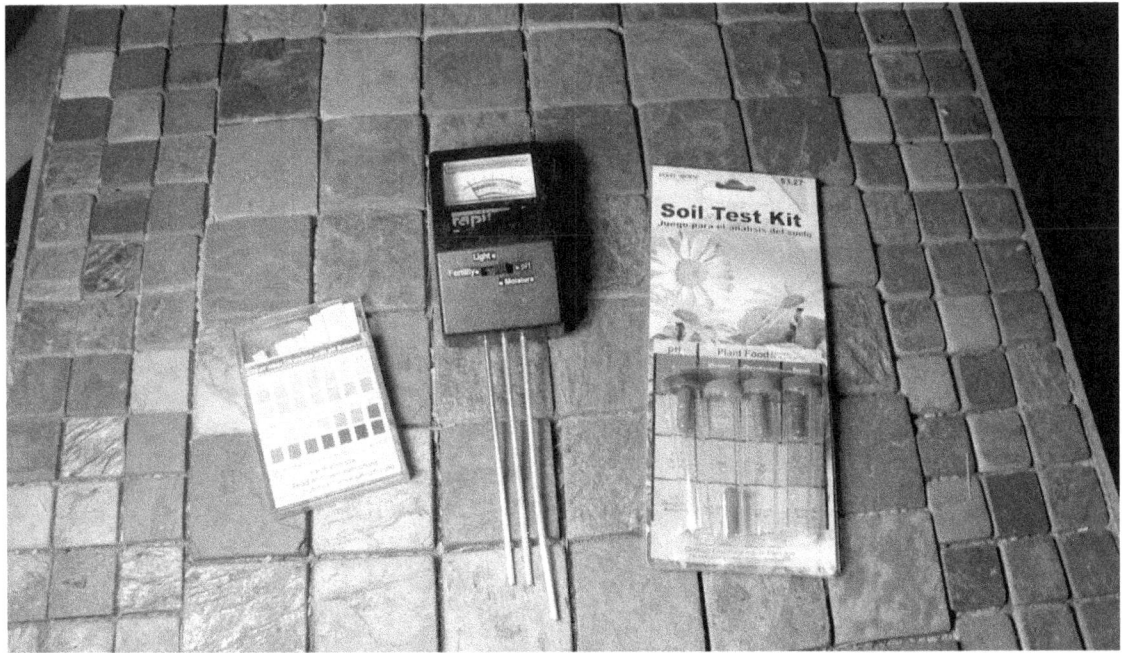

This means you will have to check the pH of your soil on a regular basis. There are soil test kits, pH testing meters and pH test strips used for medical purposes. All work the same for testing soil. I recommend you use a meter but also purchase two-color pH strips to test the meter.

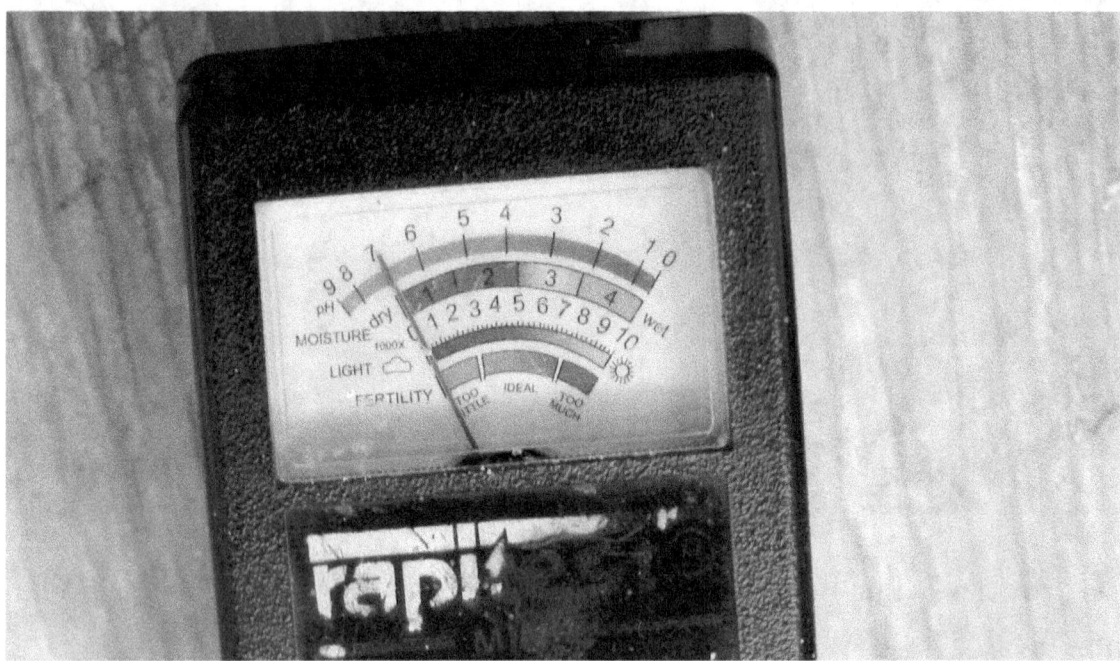

You will find the pH meter the easiest to use but always test it with something else, like the pH test strips to make sure the reading is accurate.

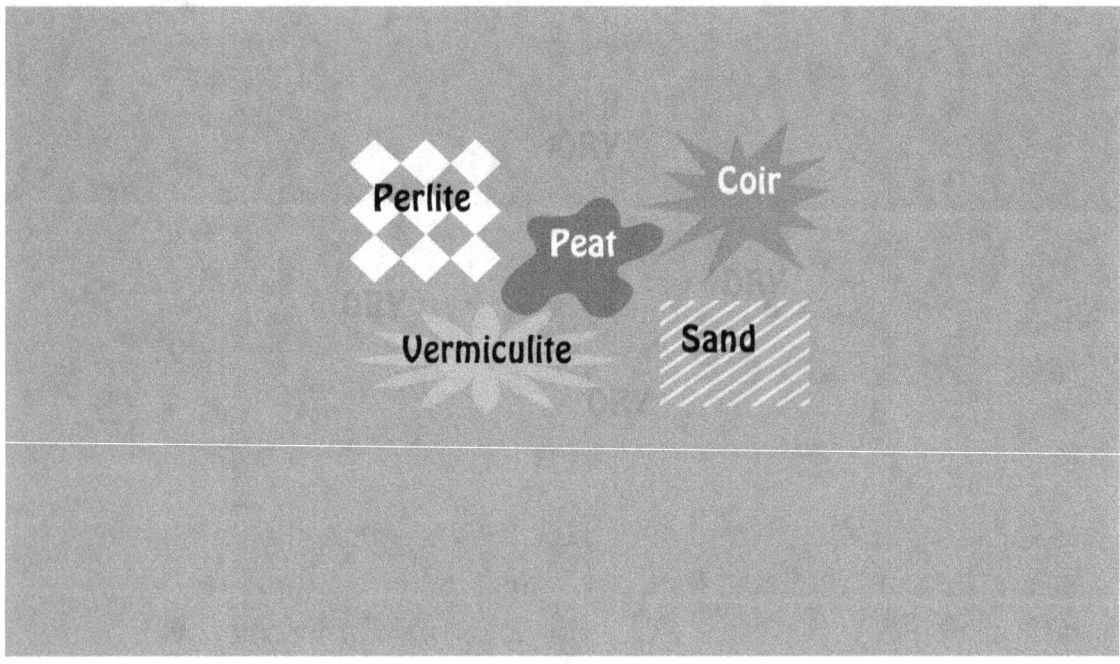

It is also important to keep in mind that the soil needs to be moist for the pH meter to read accurately. If your Coir, Peat and Vermiculite have absorbed water but it is dry between the ingredients you will get a false high reading on pH.

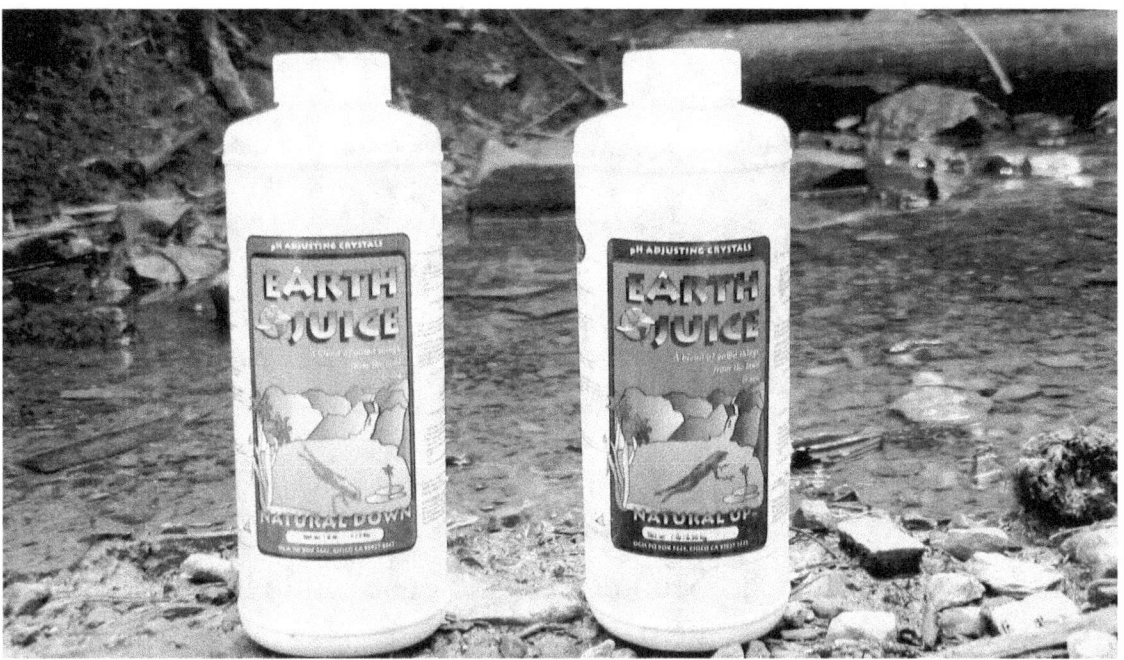

If, on the other hand you get a high reading and the soil is moist you can adjust the soil pH by adding either Natural Up or Natural Down. I use primarily Natural (pH) down which is actually vitamin C. A little goes a long way and it will not take much to lower the pH to 6.0. Natural Down is forgiving and it is easy to make corrections if you go too low. I recommended having both Natural Up and Natural Down on hand to adjust pH.

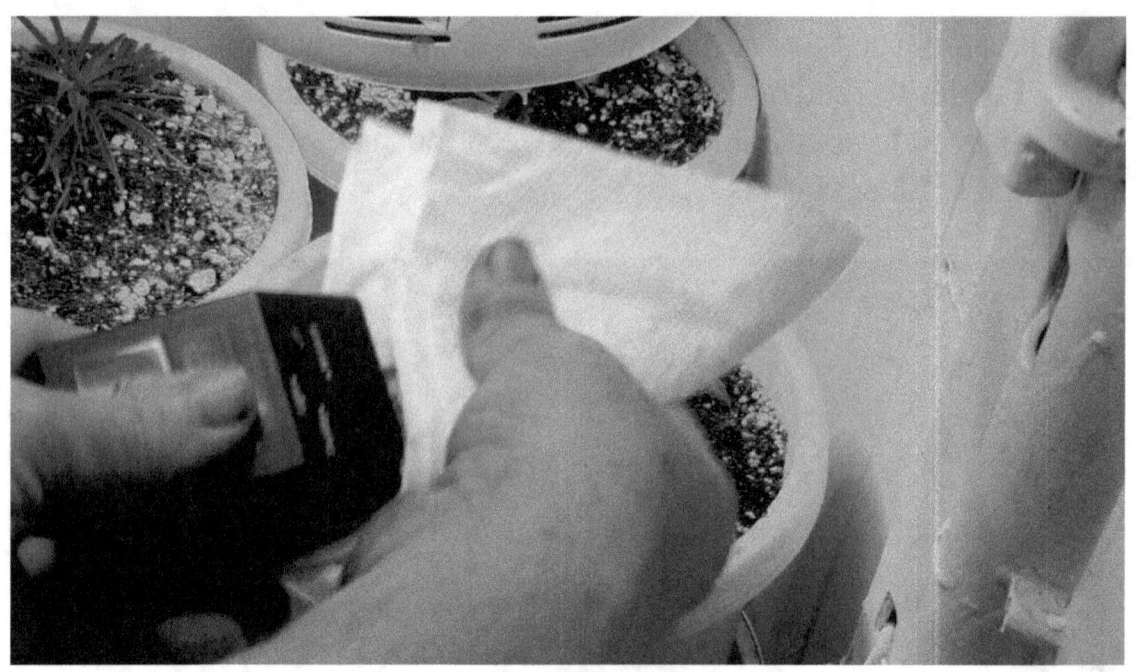

When using a meter to measure pH always make sure that you wipe off the probes after use. They won't work as well if they become corroded. And if they do become corroded use sandpaper to take off the corrosion and restore them to working order.

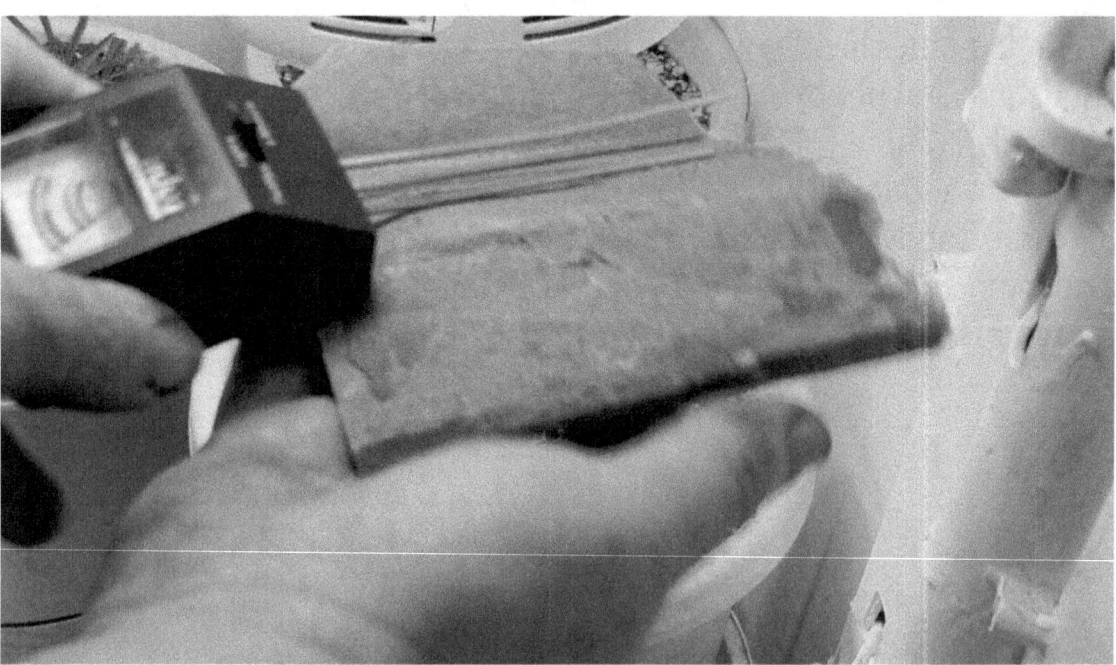

One way to start out growing your medical marijuana is to grow from seed. You can find places that sell seed on the internet at our website: http://learntogrowmedicalmarijuana.com
Will have links for buying seed. I ordered seed from the UK and was very happy with it for the most part.

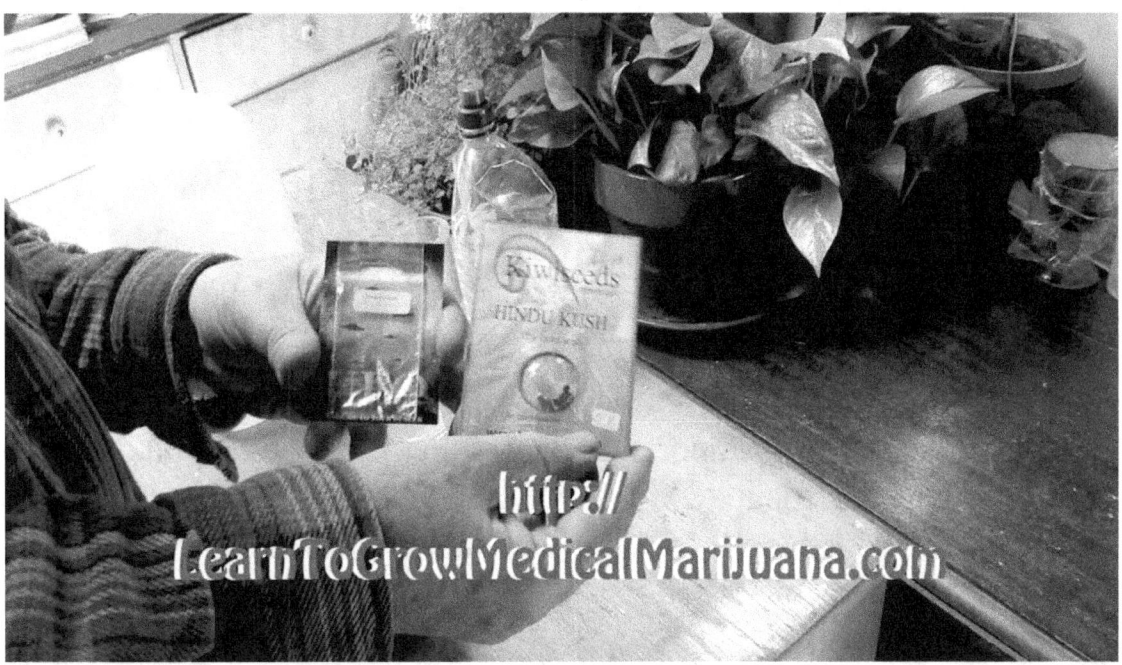

Do order more than one variety of seed. I found my favorite marijuana plant, iced grapefruit (Iced grapefruit is inexpensive, potent, and very easy to grow and clone.), after some other seeds failed and one seed that did great a Church plant, turned out to be male.

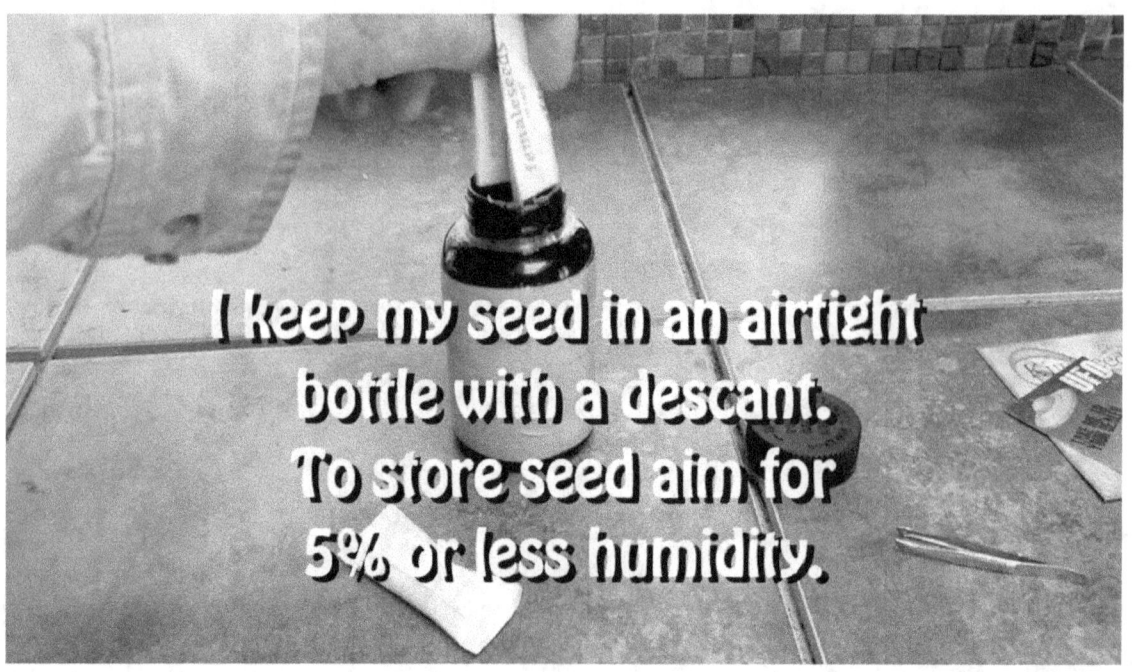

I keep my seed in an airtight bottle with a descant. To store seed aim for 5% or less humidity.

When you get seed it is important to store them properly if you don't intend to plant them right away. A container with a desiccant package will help keep your seeds at 5% or less humidity which will keep them fresh the longest.

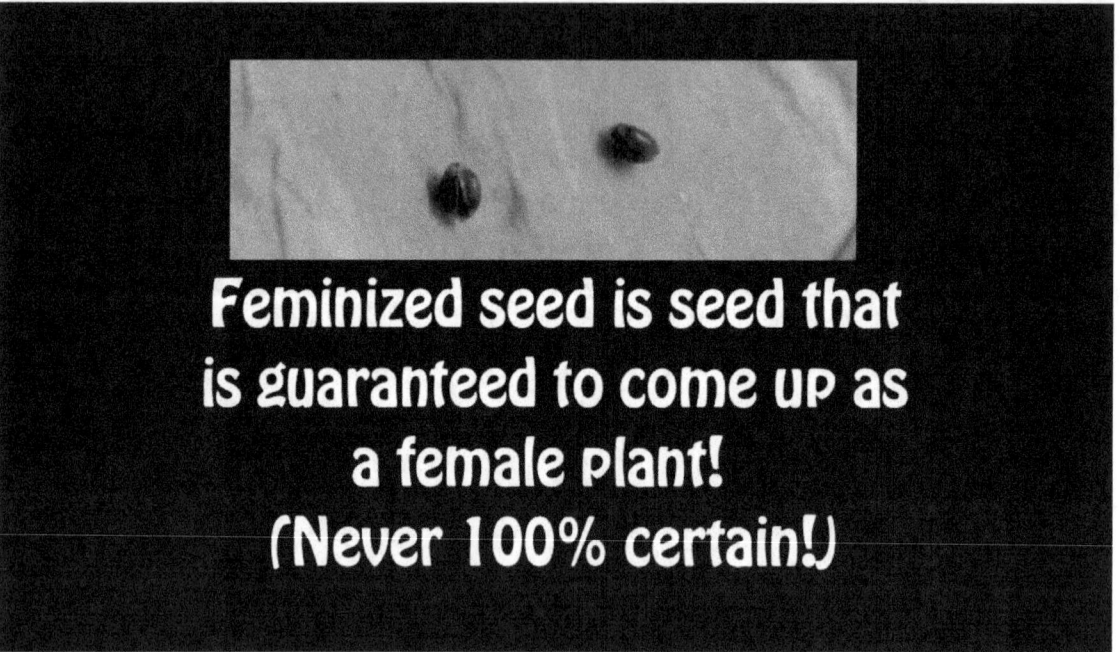

Feminized seed is seed that is guaranteed to come up as a female plant! (Never 100% certain!)

In order to have an ongoing supply of medical marijuana we grow only feminized seed and or clones. Feminized seed is seed that is induced to grow from a female plant that should produce female plants. Feminized seed is never 100%.

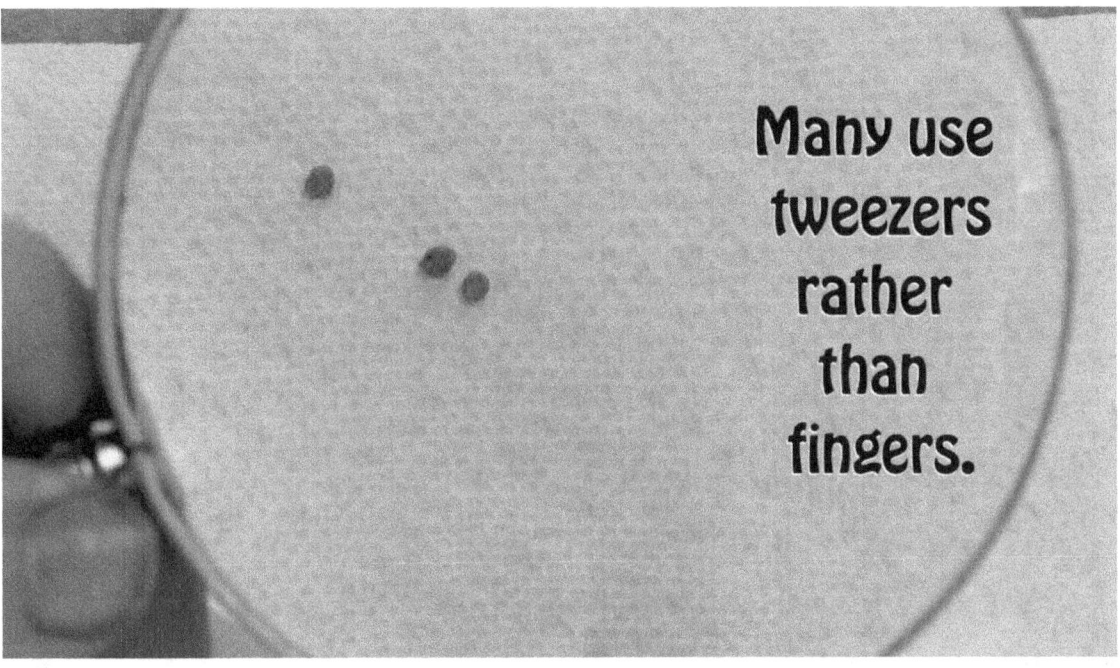

Many growers insist on using tweezers to pick up seed. I wash with an alcohol gel and do pick up my seeds by hand-though tweezers are safer.

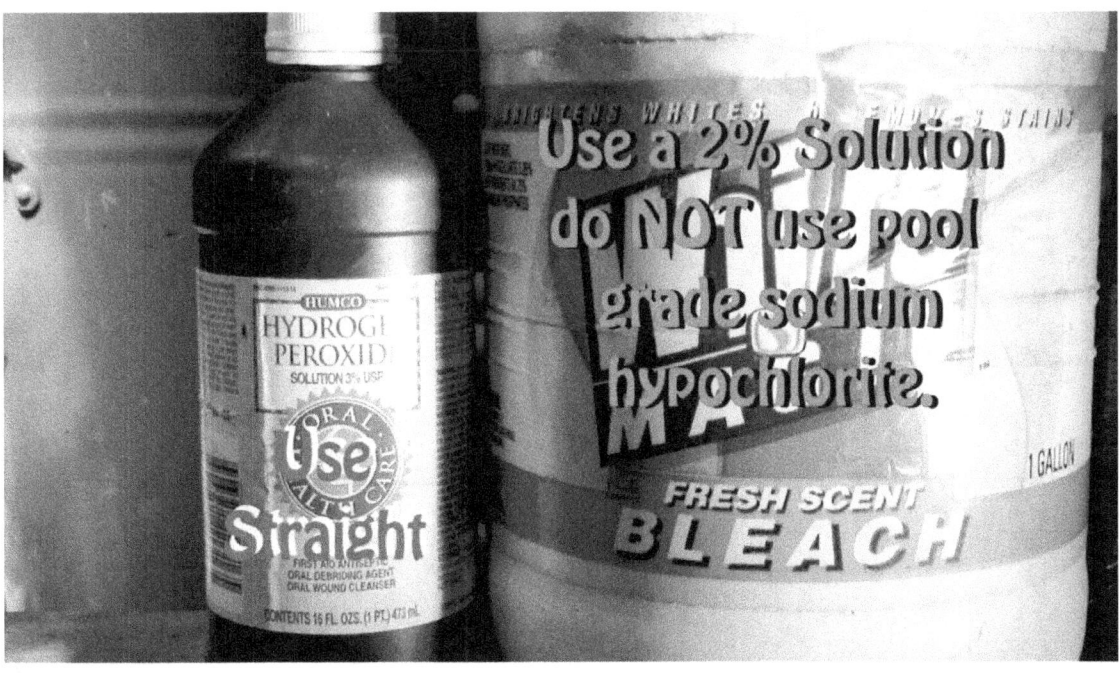

If you believe your seed may have been exposed to fungi, etc., you can treat the seed with first aid kit grade hydrogen peroxide or a 2% solution of household bleach. (Do not use pool sodium hypochlorite as pool formulas can be very strong.)

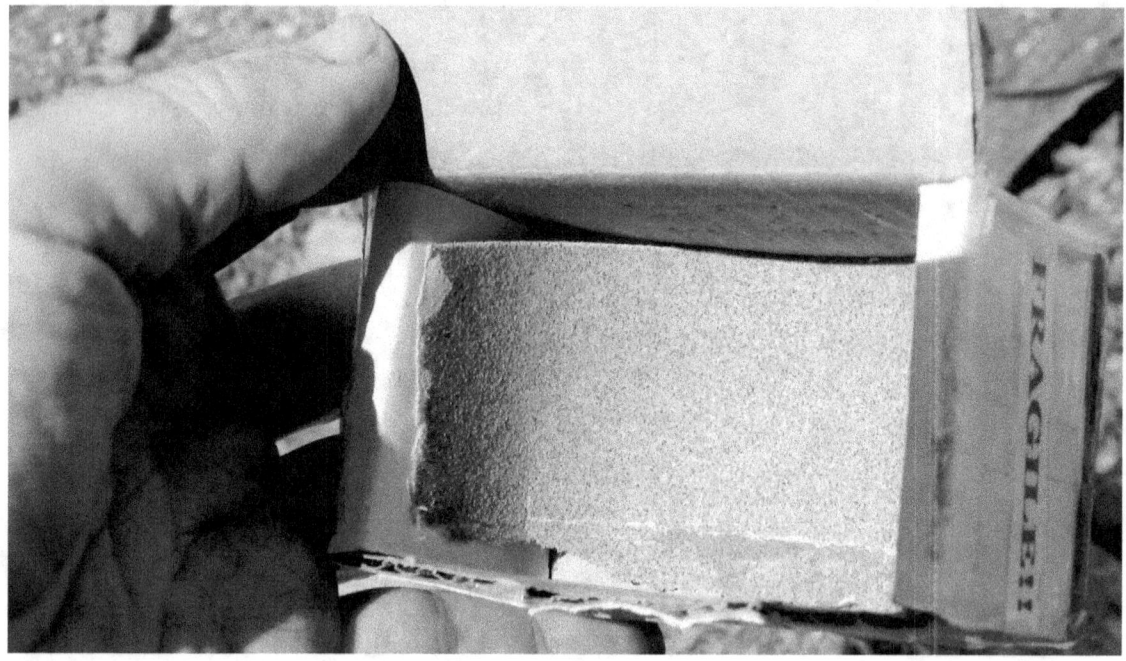

Although a sandpaper box is not necessary, I have always have quicker success when using the box. A cardboard box is fitted with sandpaper inside. Seeds are placed inside and shaken for 5 minutes. The abrasions on the seed's skin help the seed soak faster.

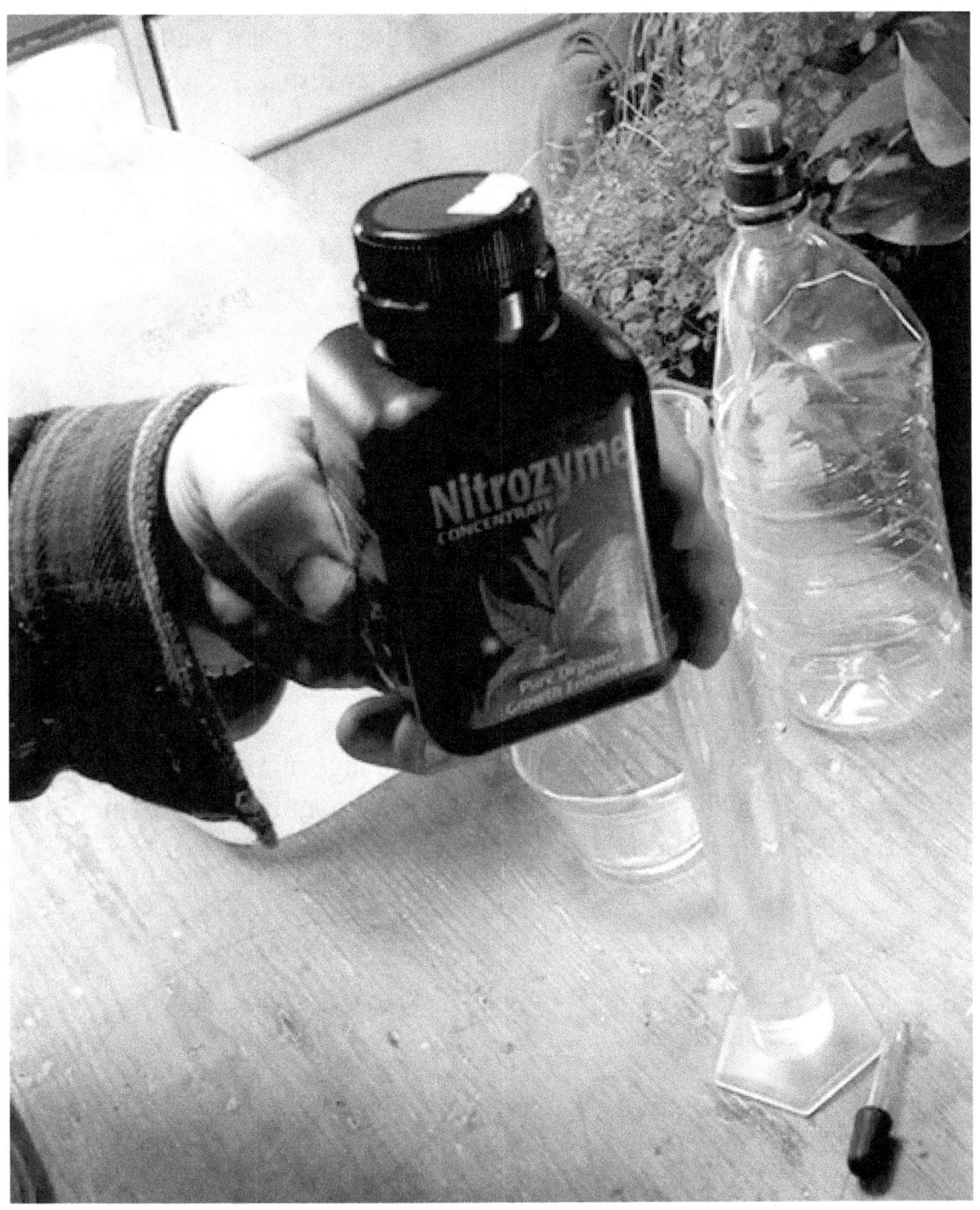

To soak my seed I use a 2% solution of Nitrosyme. Nitrosyme is imported from the UK. If you have trouble finding it you can use Liquid Seaweed instead. The Nitrosyme is one of my favorite growing aids, as it increases growth and reduces budding in my iced-grapefruit from 8 weeks to 7. I don't use much of the seed soaking mixture and usually put 1 ml of nitrosyme in 50 mls of water. When I am done with the soak I dilute the remaining Nitrosyme by adding 3 parts water and use the resulting .5% solution as a fertilizer or foliar fertilizer.

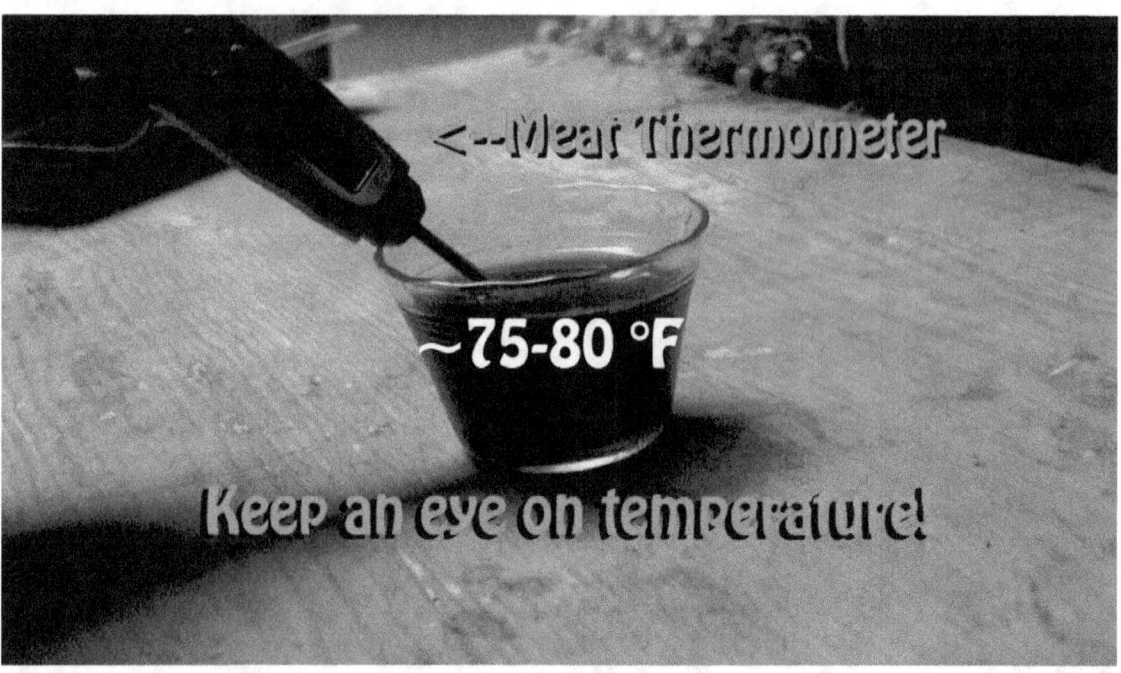

A warm temperature in your soak will help things along. Anything from 70 °F to 80 °F will work fine. I find it convenient to use a meat thermometer to measure soil and liquid temperatures.

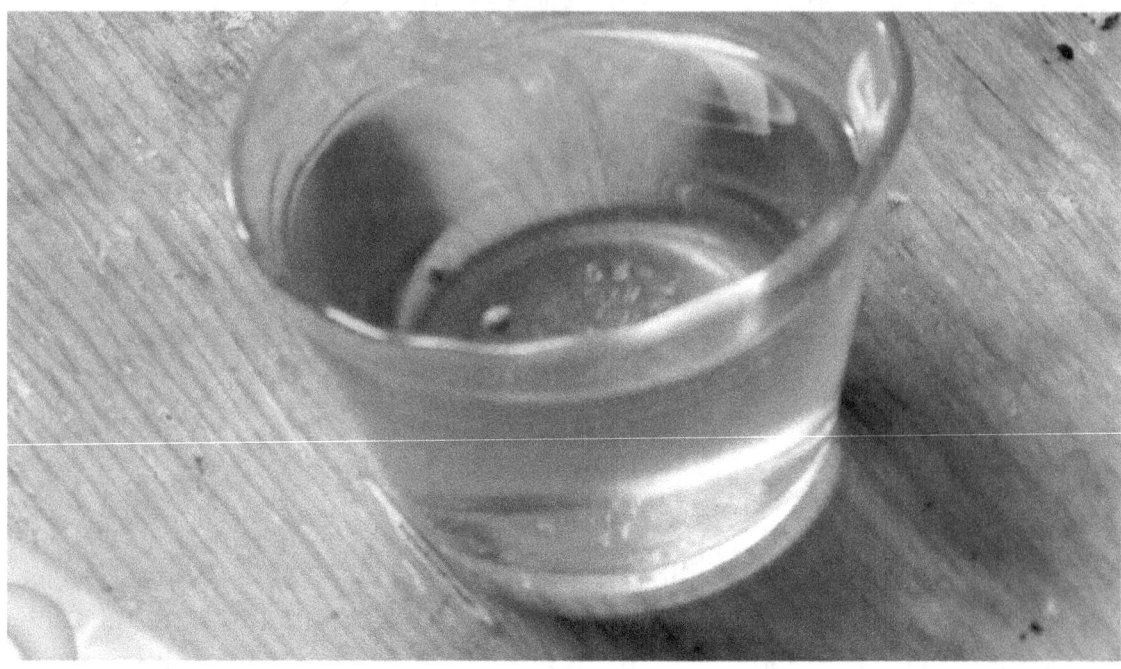

You can use plain distilled water if you like. Soak your seed overnight. Viable seeds will sink. If a seed doesn't sink tap it to knock off any air bubbles. If it still doesn't sink it is probably not going to grow.

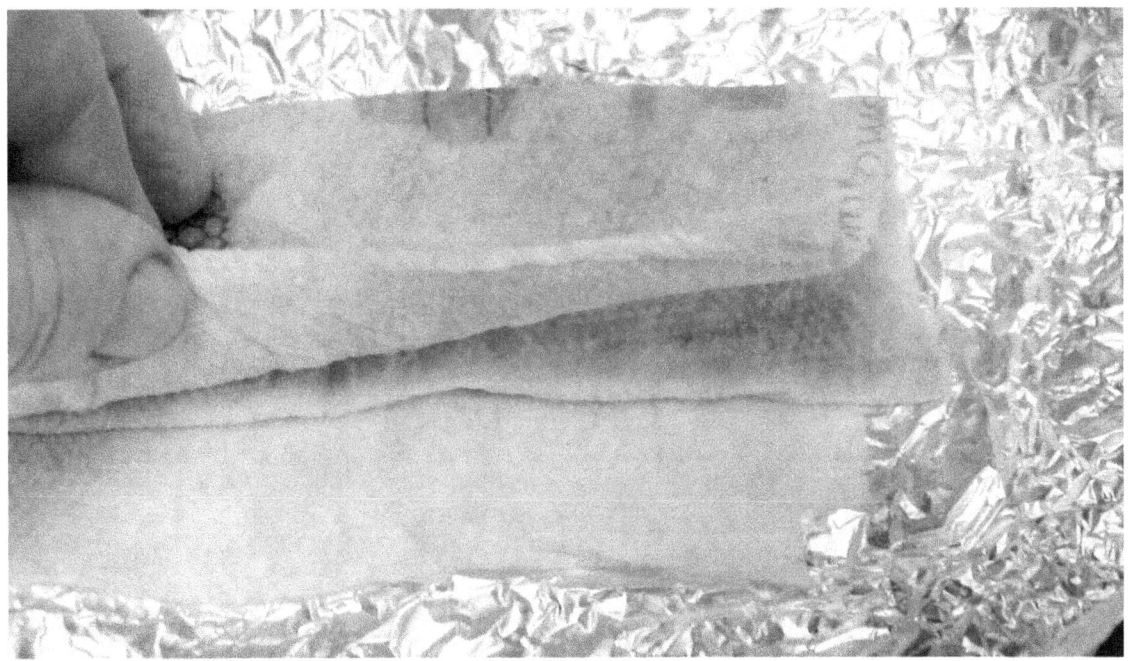

Wrap the seed in a paper towel wetted with your 2% nitrosyme solution (before diluting it). Don't make the paper towel so wet that the seeds drown. The towel should be damp not wet. Wring it out if need be. Wrap the paper towel in a piece of aluminum foil so that it is light tight and put it in a warm place overnight.

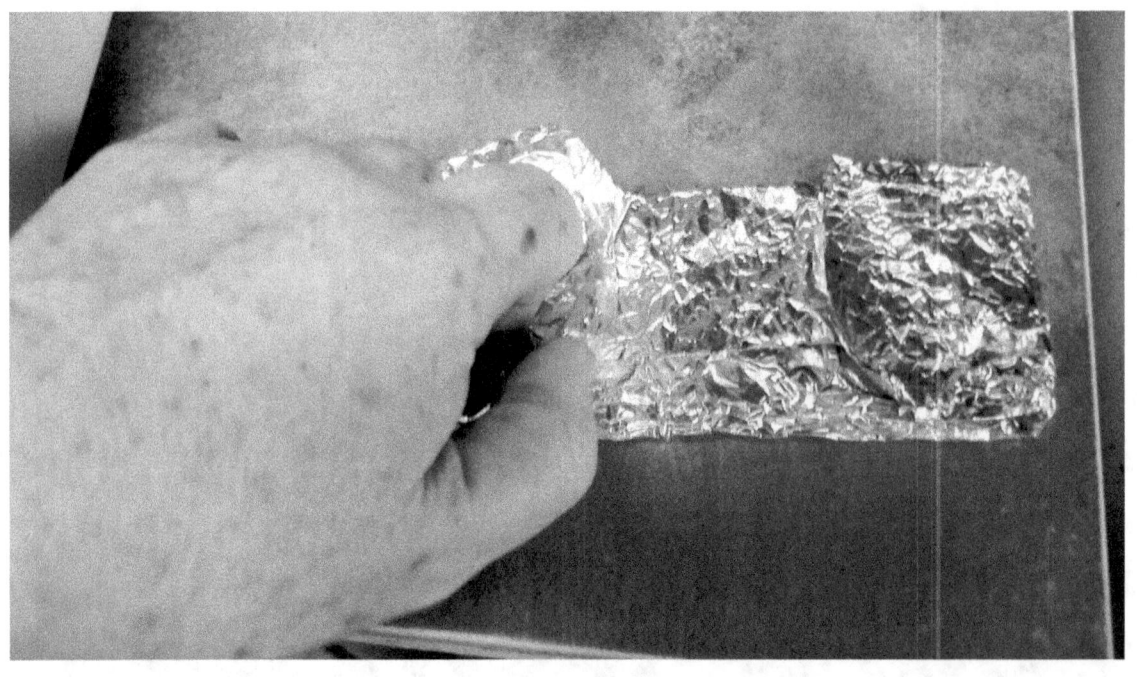

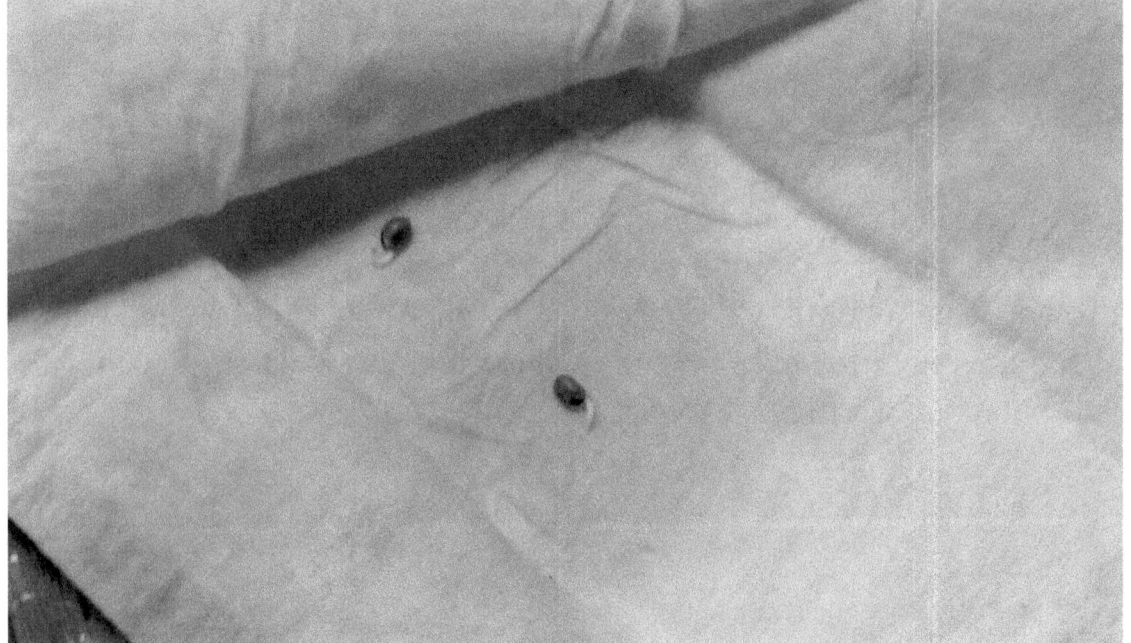

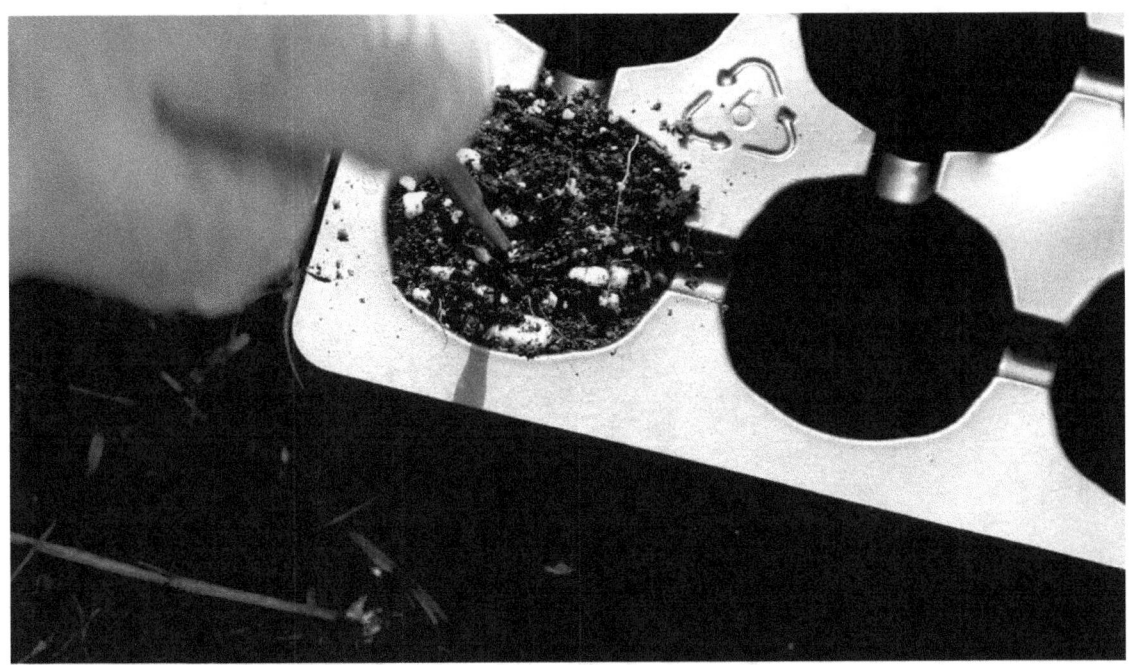

To plant poke a hole in the soil and then with tweezers plant the seedling sprout down.

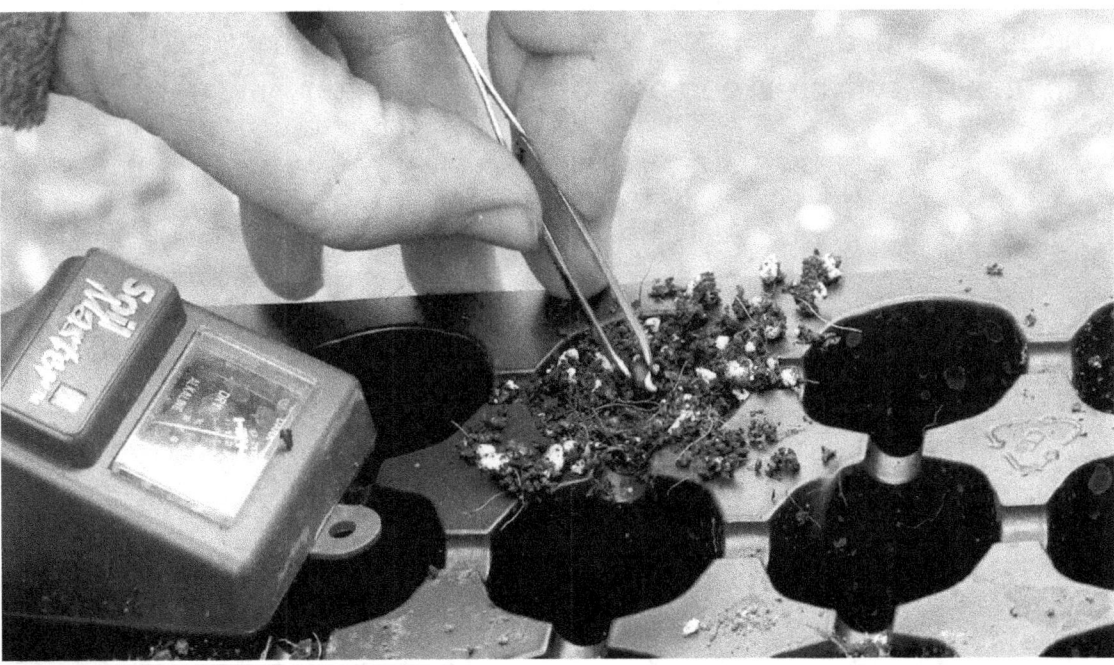

Every time I have used the sandpaper box and the Nitrosyme the seeds have sprouted in the paper towel by the next day. I have planted seeds without the soak or sandpaper box and they took 3 to 5 days to sprout.

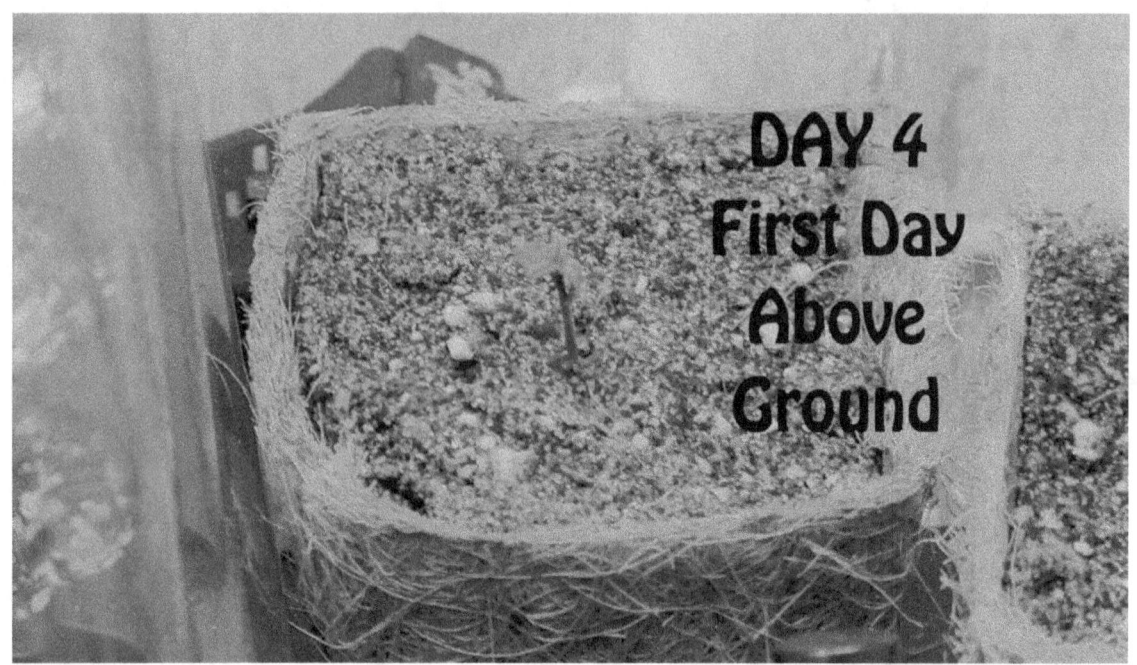

DAY 4
First Day
Above
Ground

I planted the seedlings in coir pots with my soil mix and in jiffy pots which I expanded with a .5% Nitrosyme solution.   I have had success with both my soil mix in coir pots or peat pots, and in jiffy pots.

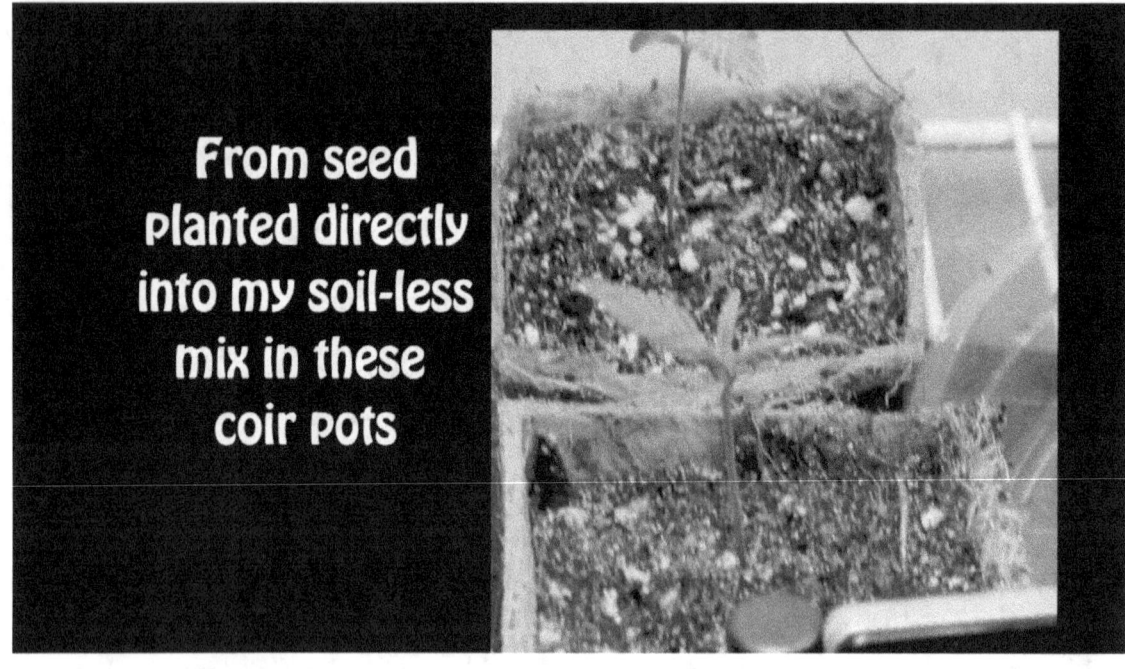

From seed planted directly into my soil-less mix in these coir pots

I have used humidity domes for seedlings but no longer use them. I found that once seedlings come up, higher humidity hurts rather than helps. If you do use a humidity dome for seedlings make sure you take them out as soon as they break ground.

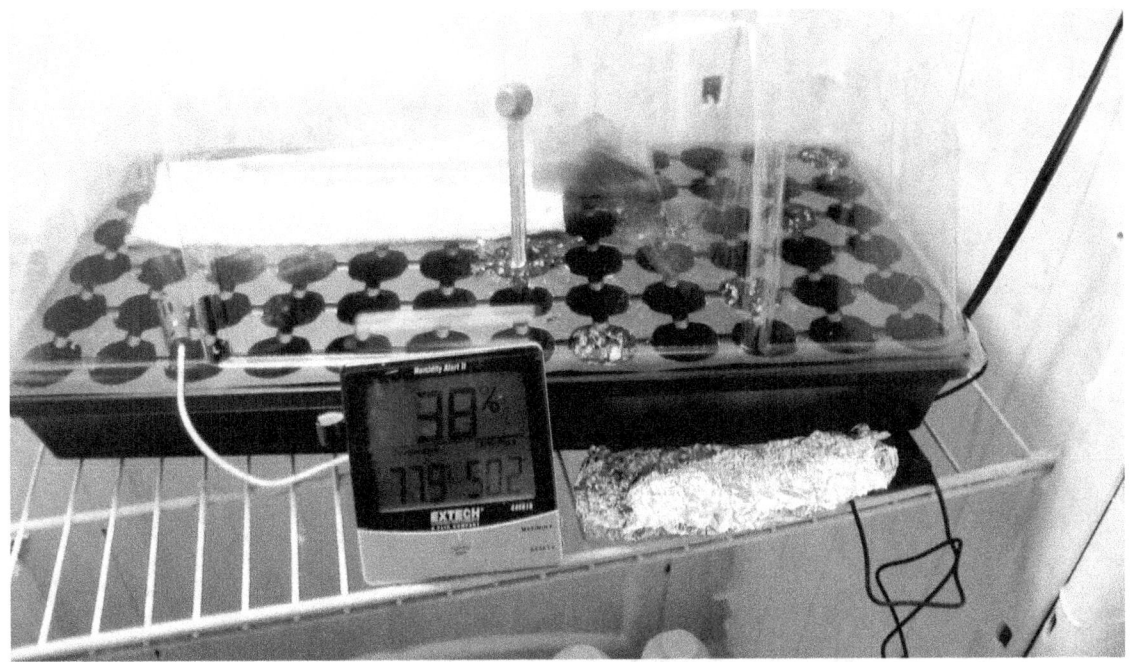

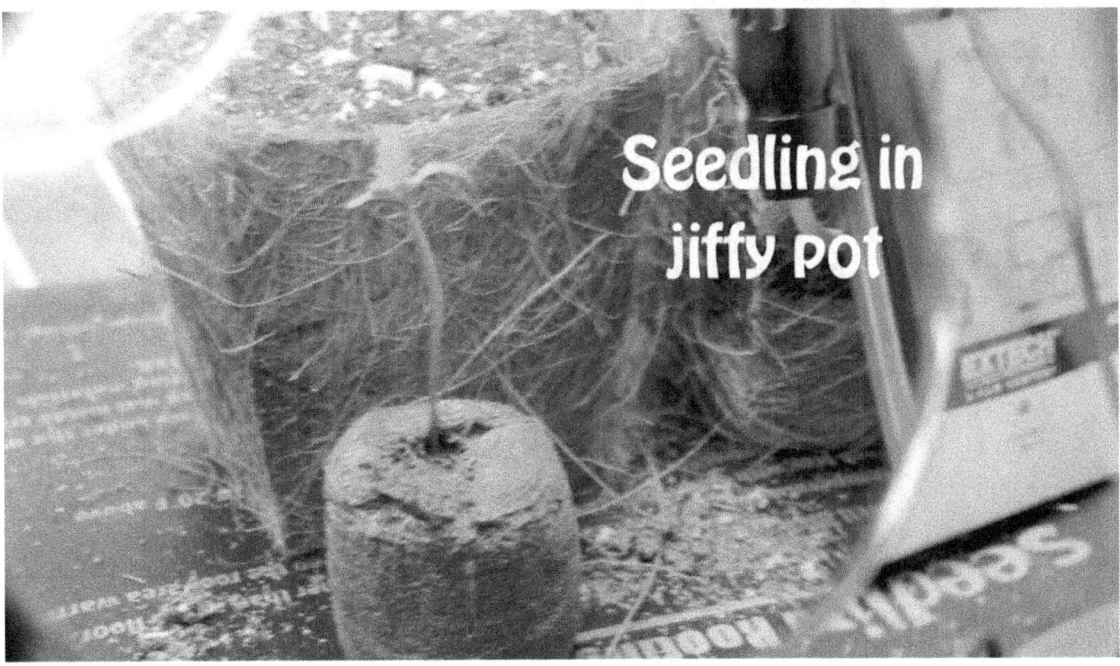

Seedling in jiffy pot

Expandable jiffy pots do work quite well and take up less room initially than coir or peat pots. I soak them in .5% Nitrosyme until they expand.

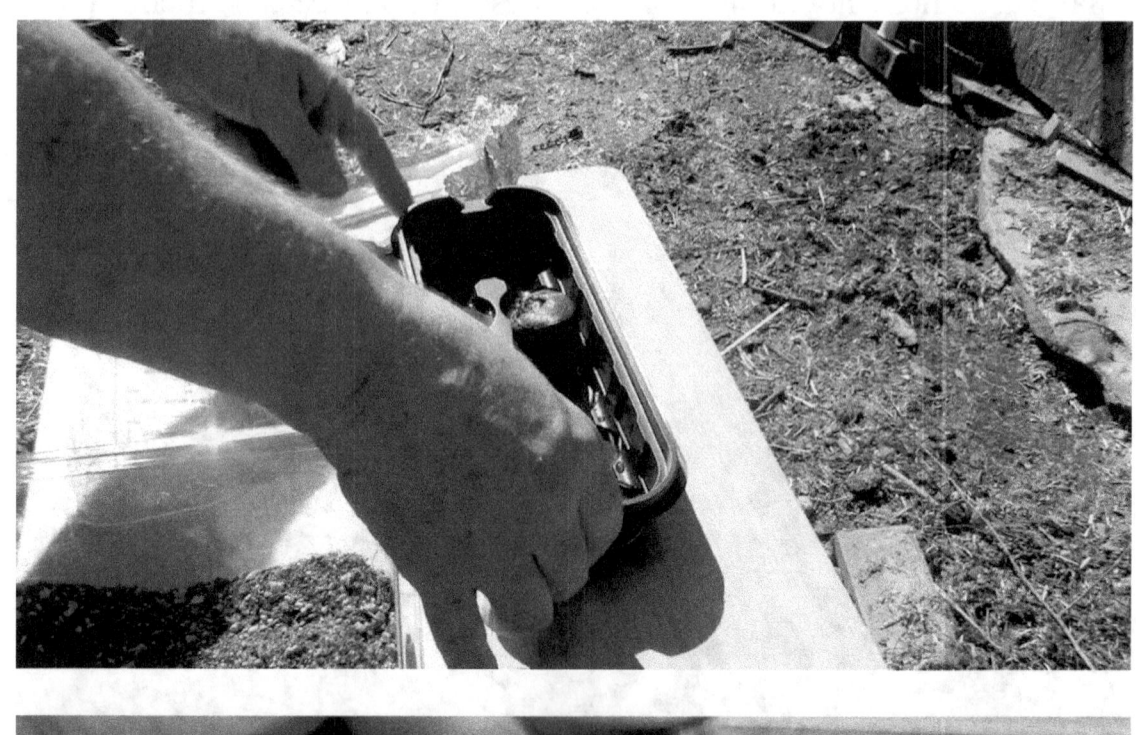

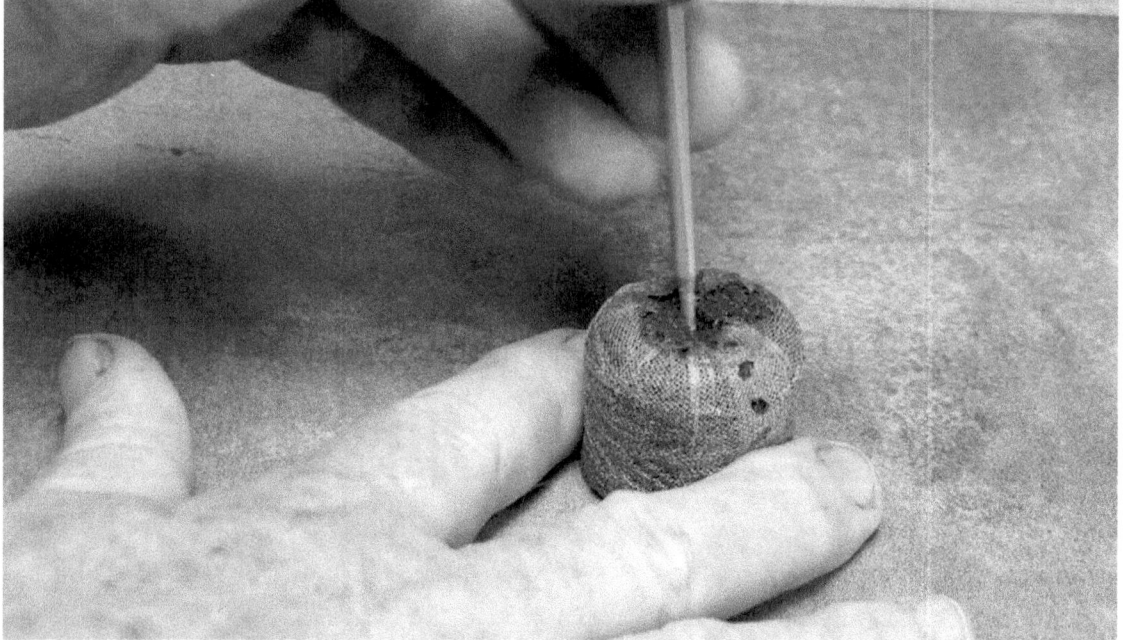

To plant poke a hole as you would with soil and simply insert the seedling sprout down.

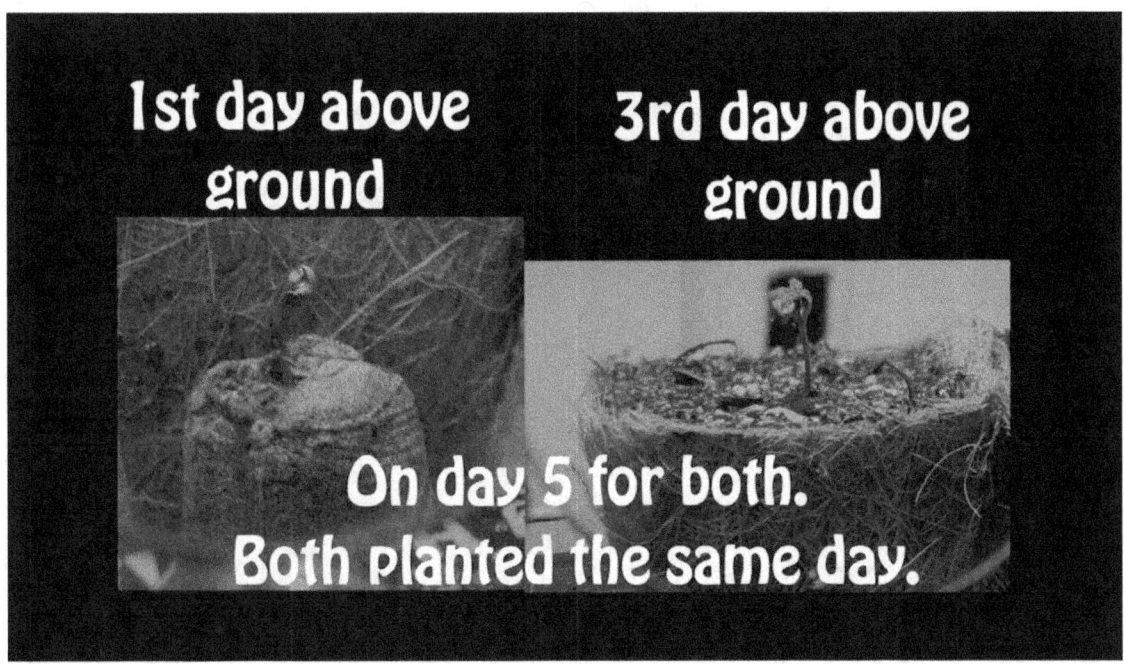

A comparison of coir pot with my soil and a jiffy pot show pretty much the same growth on the 5th day for both seedlings.

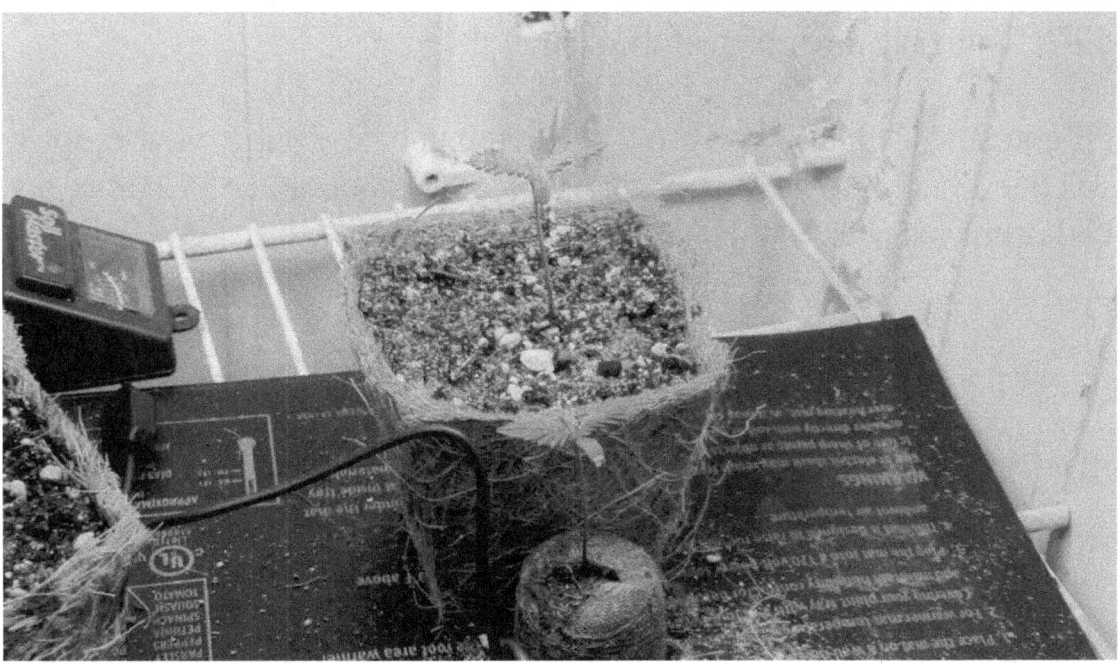

If you have a heating pad, perhaps one that came with a humidity dome, use it for your seedlings. They will growth faster with warmer soil.

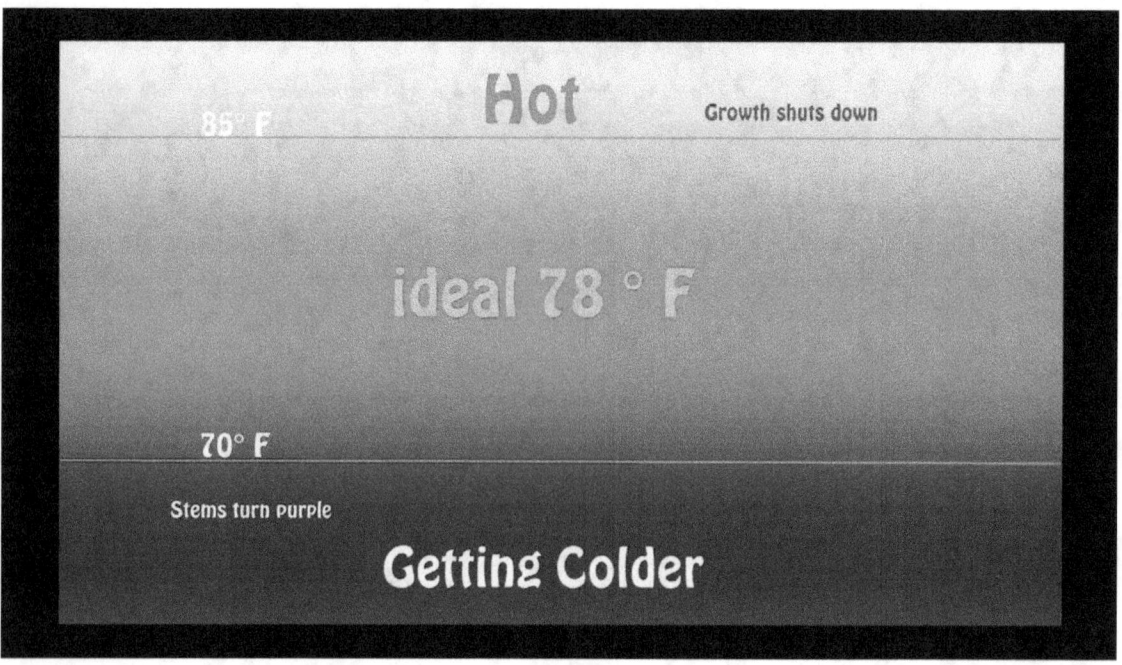

The ideal temperature for your medical marijuana is about 78° F higher temperatures than 85° F , and lower than 70° F do not enhance growth. I have had my plants room temperature go down to 59° F with only a purpling of the stem.

Of course what plants you grow will determine how hardy your crop will be. I have had great success with Iced Grapefruit, and Church, but had problems with both Hindu Kush and Bubba Kush.

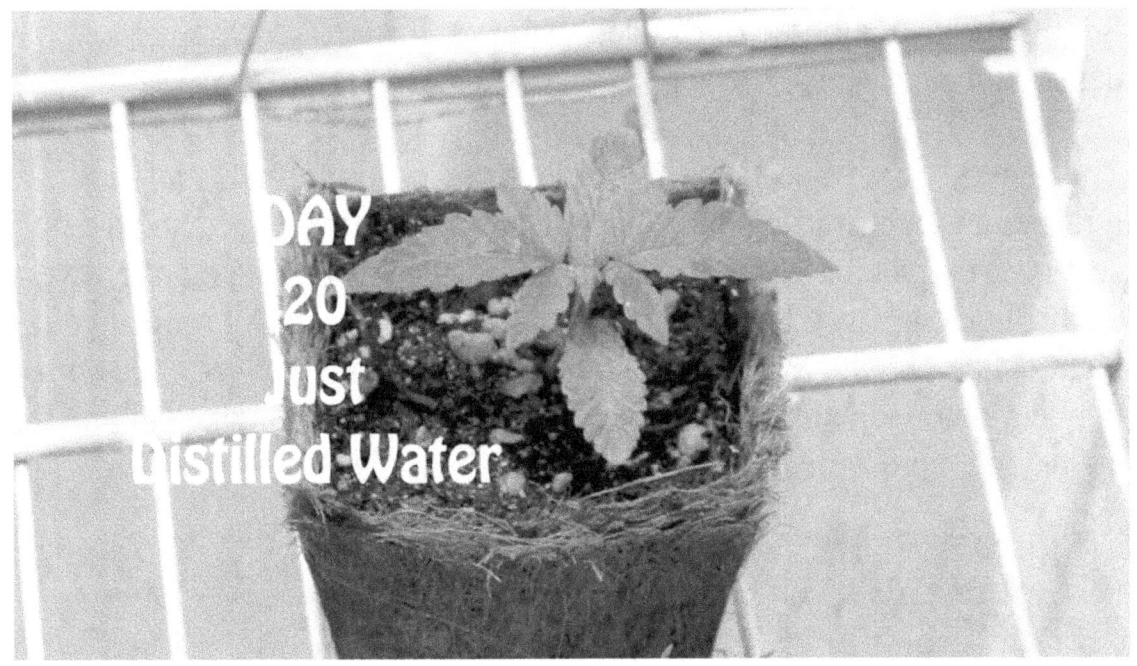

With any new seedlings do not use anything but water for the first three weeks. Adding fertilizer before then will burn the leaf tips.

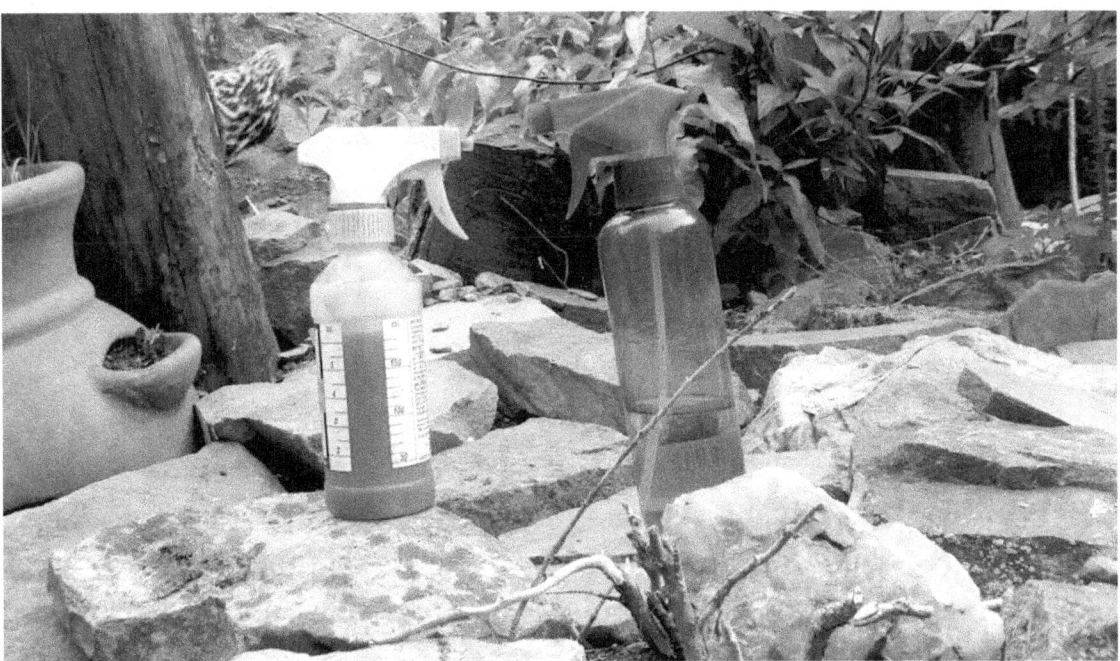

Do keep spray bottles on hand. My blue one is distilled water. I use this when non-foliar (that is normal) fertilizer splashes on plants leaves. Fertilizer can kill leaves when applied directly, as can other chemicals.

So always have a bottle of distilled water on hand to wash off any unintentional splashes.

The second bottle I used for my .5% nitrosyme spray that is a foliar fertilizer and which I do spray on all leaves every day. Spraying the seaweed extract increases shoot growth as well as overall plant growth. Again, liquid seaweed can be used instead of nitrosyme. I may have been enticed by the lure of a product imported from the UK. I have noticed water solutions of liquid seaweed do get a sulfur smell after awhile that nitrosyme does not get.

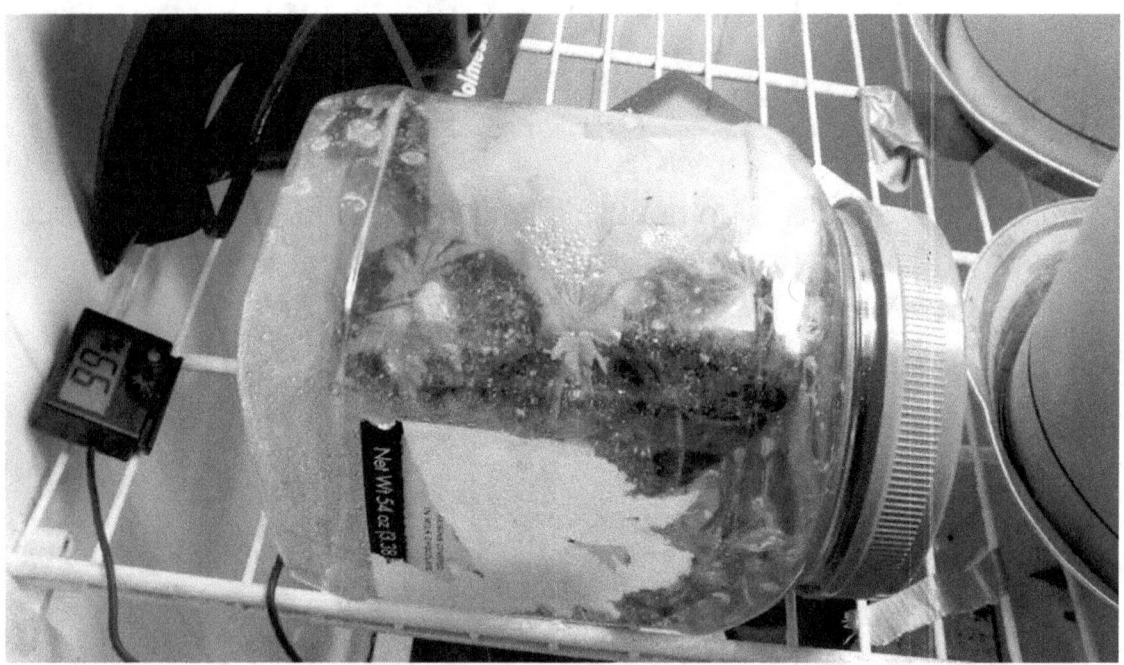

Although seedlings are a great way to grow marijuana starting from seed is a slow process and may take 5 months or more to harvest a crop. When you seed in a seed listing that a plant flowers in 8 weeks. This mean in 8 weeks of being in a bloom shed. The plant will most likely need two months at least before that to grow and mature.

On the other hand a clone, a cutting which has been taking from a larger plant called a mother plant[1], is already as old as the mother, already if old enough--sexually mature, and can produce a crop months earlier than you can with seed.

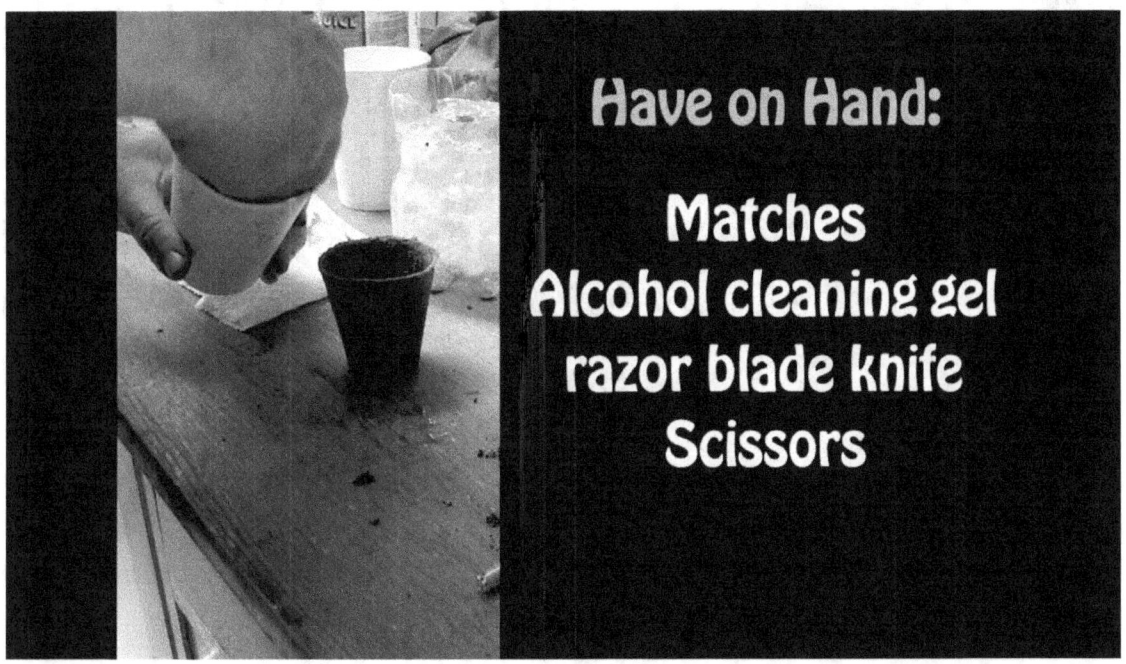

To make a clone you will need matches and/or alcohol cleaning gel, a razor sharp knife, scissors, distilled water or nitrosyme, a humidity dome of some kind, a jiffy pot or a peat or coir pot with our soil-less mix, and a cloning agent.

----

[1] Mother plants, by the way, can be male or female, however, most of us will only be using females as mother plants.

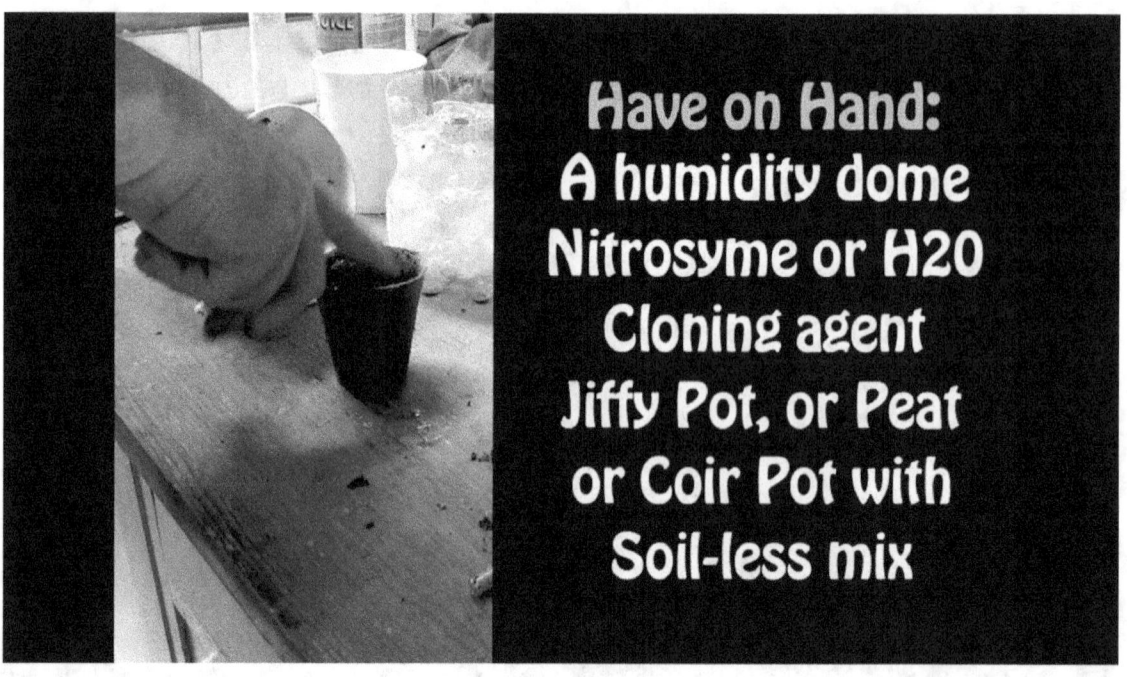

Have on Hand:
A humidity dome
Nitrosyme or H20
Cloning agent
Jiffy Pot, or Peat
or Coir Pot with
Soil-less mix

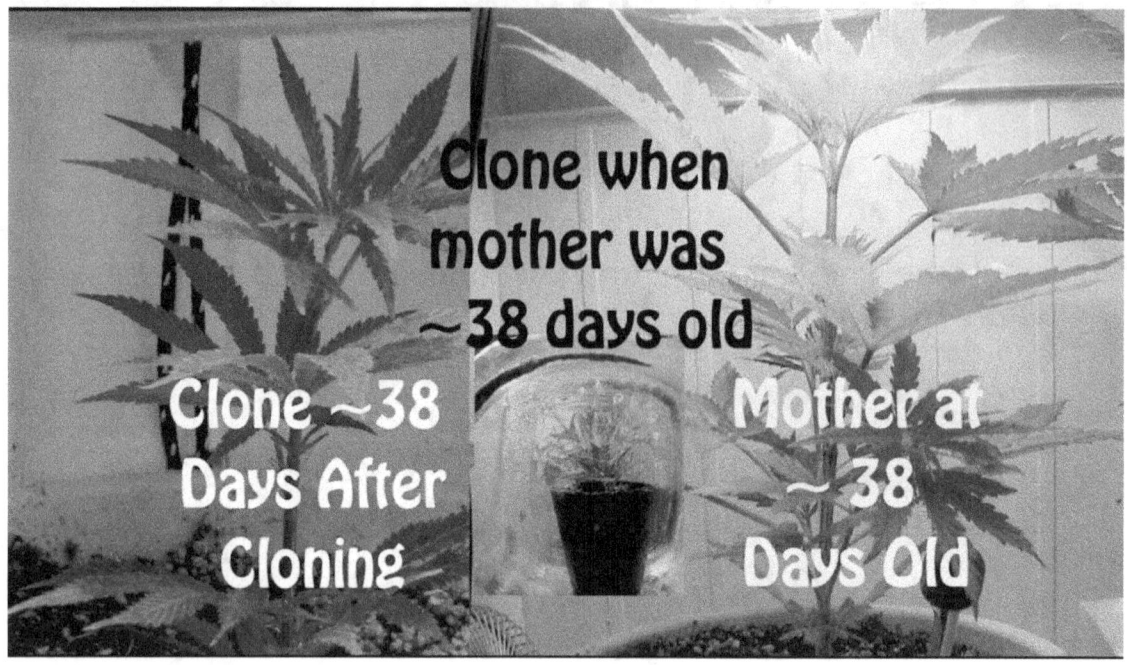

Clone when mother was ~38 days old

Clone ~38 Days After Cloning

Mother at ~38 Days Old

Clones tend to be almost duplicates of the mother plant as photo comparisons of mother and clone show at the same age.

And as long as you don't unnecessarily stress the plant it should be just as female as the mother. [II]

To create a clone the first thing you need to do is sterilize your scissors, of razor blade. I use matches on my Exacto knife. And on my scissor which have plastic handles I use the same 50% ethyl alcohol hand washing gel I use on my hands which sterilizes as well as cleans.

If you are using a jiffy pot you will need to soak the pot in distilled water or a .5% nitrosyme solution to expand the jiffy pot. If you are using a coir or peat pot with your soil-less mixture you should have that ready to go.

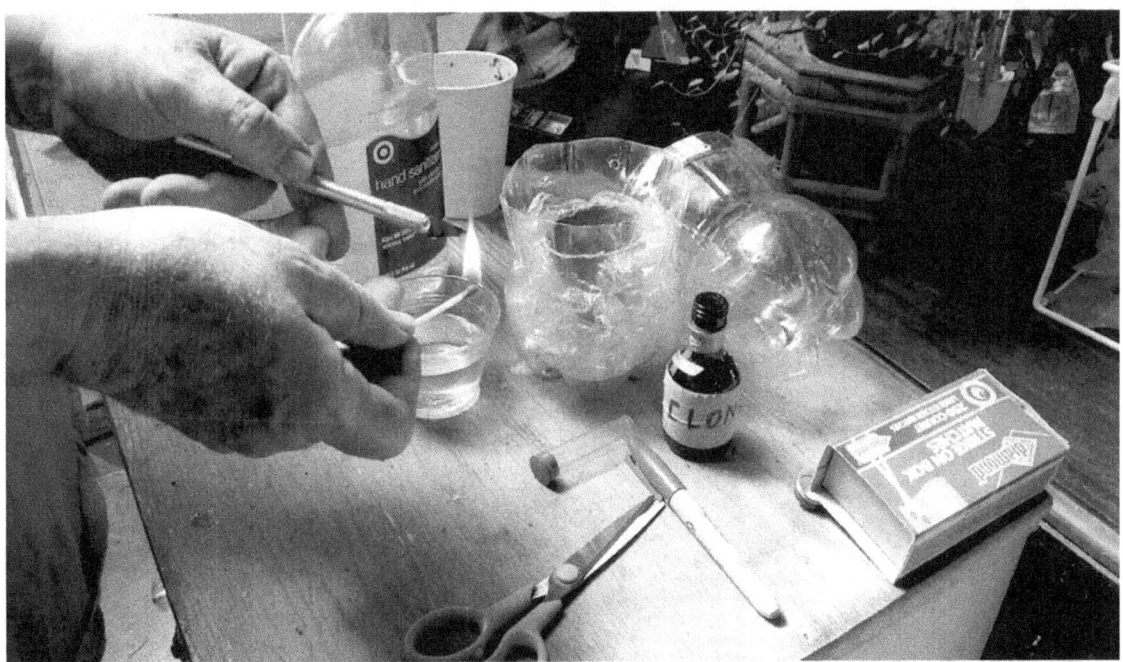

[II] Stress can cause hermaphrodites to develop. For our production of medicine we don't want male plants or even partial male plants as seed development reduces medicine development.

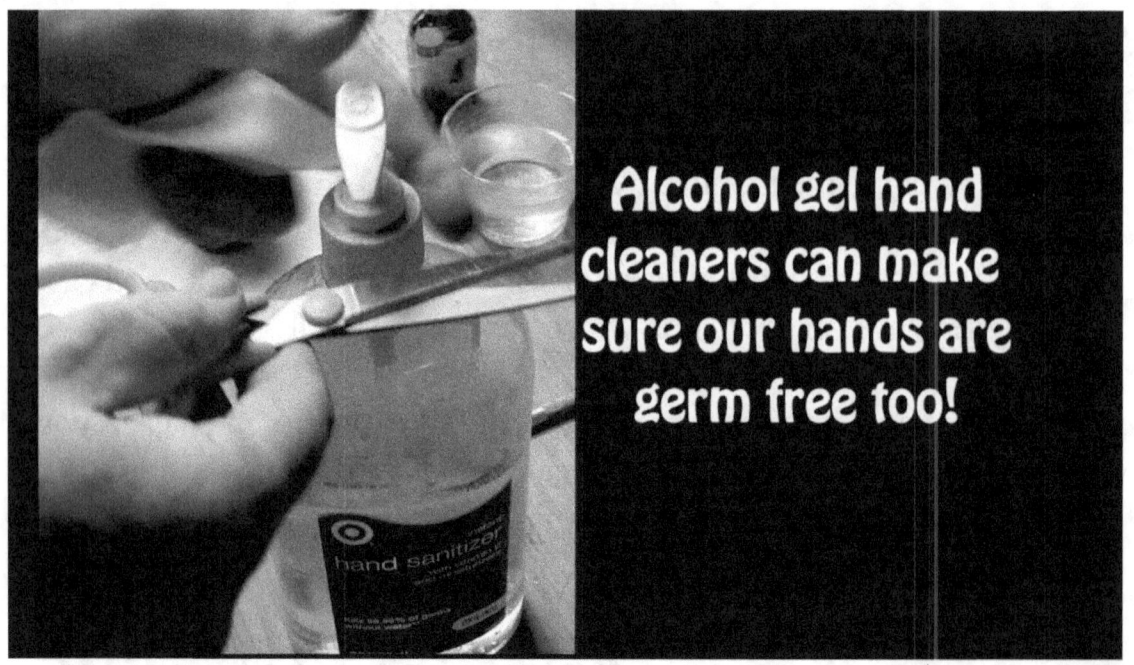

Alcohol gel hand cleaners can make sure our hands are germ free too!

Once you have everything sterilized put some distilled water or .5% Nitrosyme solution in a shallow bowl like the one in the photo above (just above the tip of the scissors in the photo.)

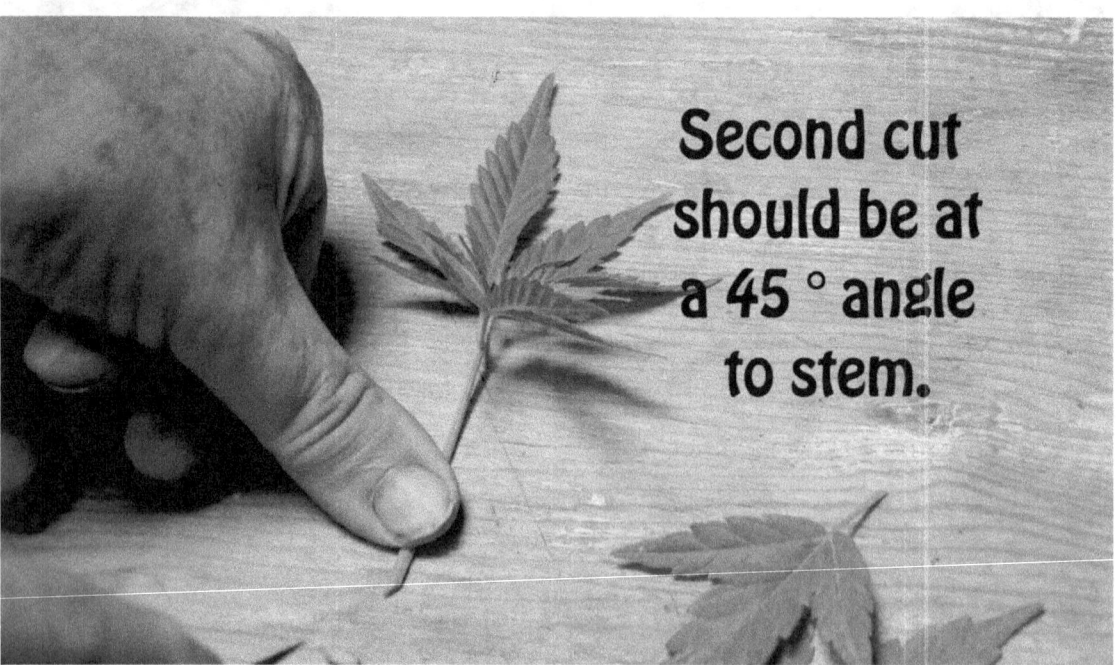

Second cut should be at a 45 ° angle to stem.

Although I am cutting here on a table so the photos show where I am cutting, I actually do the cutting underwater or under a .5% nitrosyme solution. After cutting the cutting from the plant, put the stem in your water or solution and cut again just a little further up at a 45° angle.

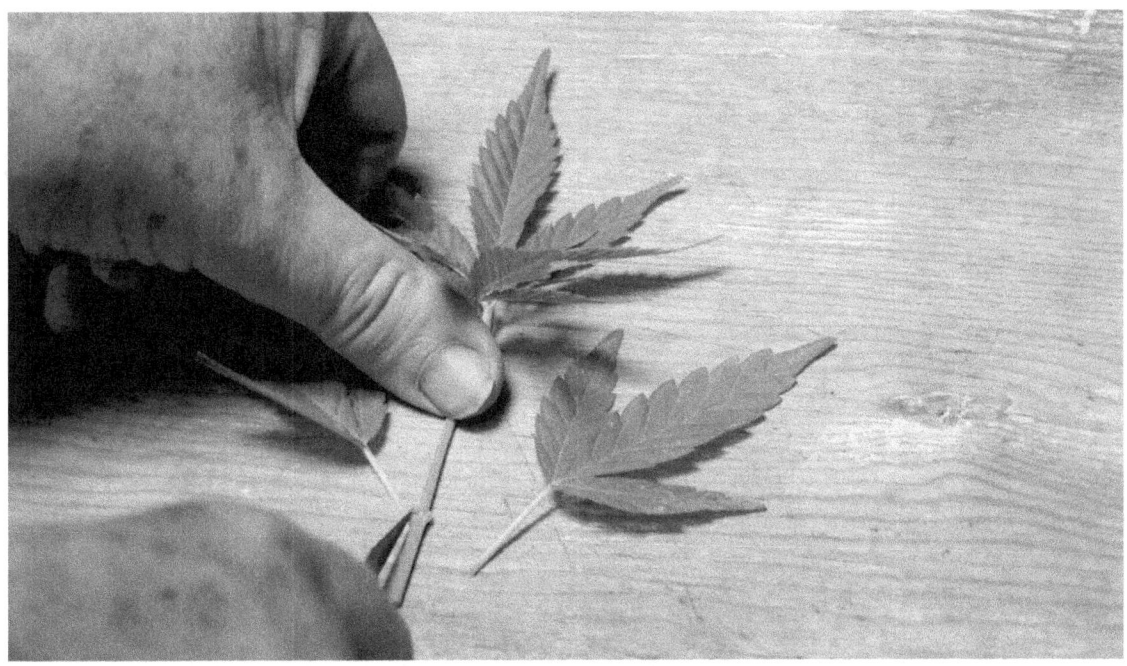

Next trim off any lower leaves. The nodes left are good sites for roots to develop.

Then, still underwater, split the stem partway up.

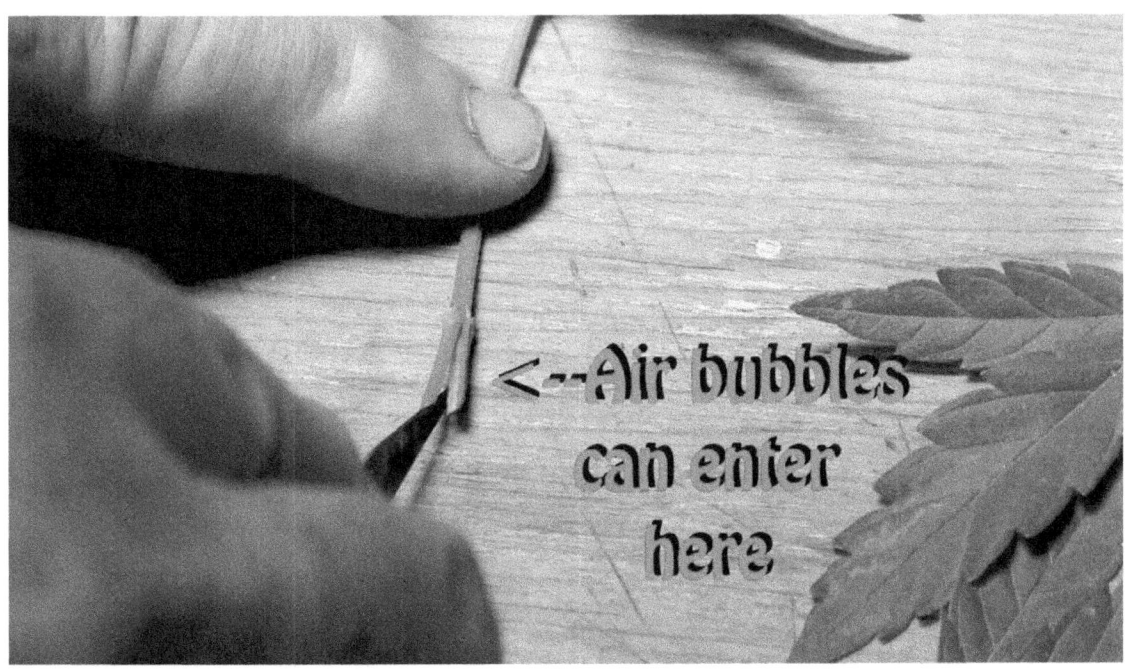

If you do this in the air, air bubbles can enter the plant , but if you do it underwater they will not.

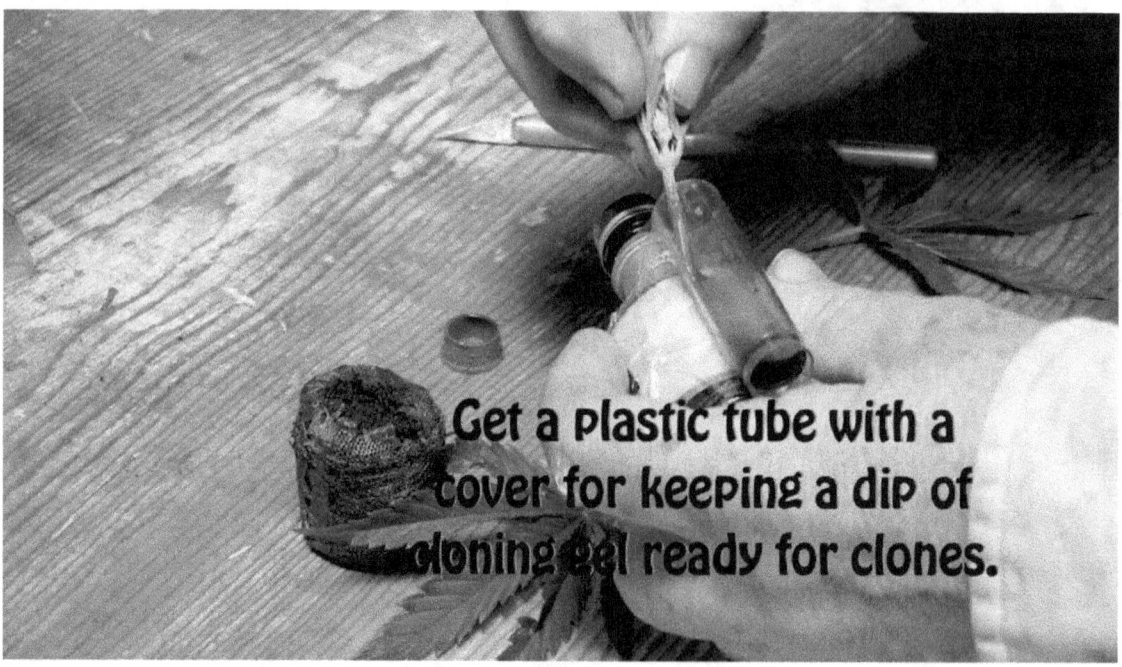

Get a plastic tube with a cover for keeping a dip of cloning gel ready for clones.

Put some cloning gel[III] in a tube and coat the stem thoroughly.

[III] Use gel not powder (which has never worked for me) or liquid. The gels coat the stems well, stay on and work. I have used Clonex with the best success, even though it is not for edible plants.

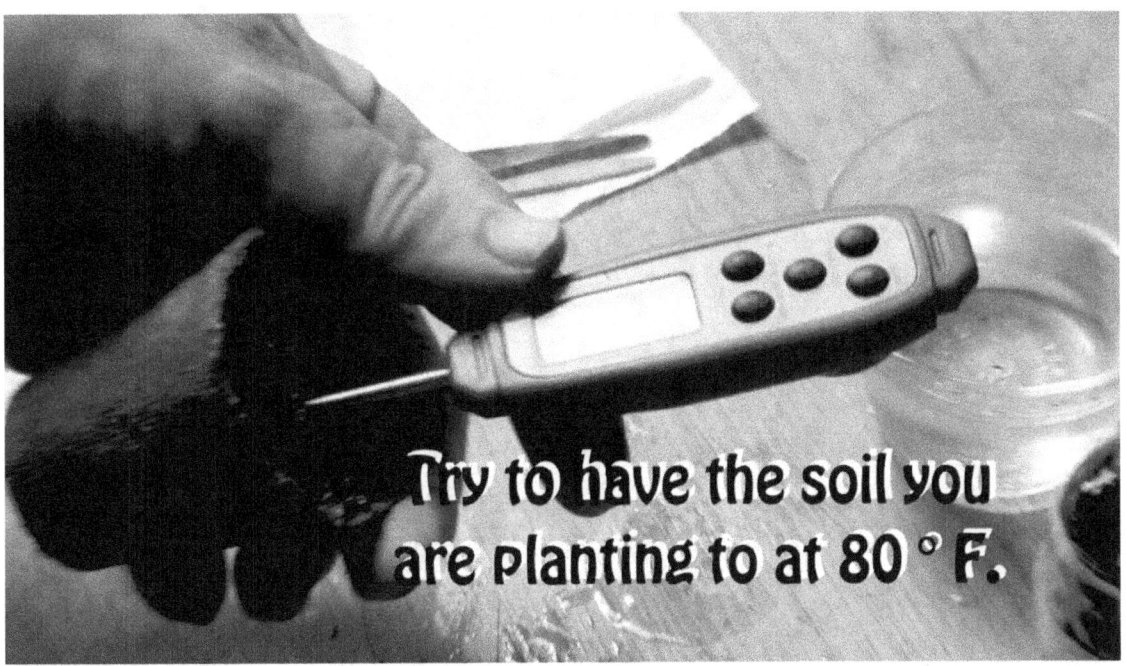

Then place the coated stem in your coir pot, peat pot, or jiffy pot. Do have the pot warm: 80° F.

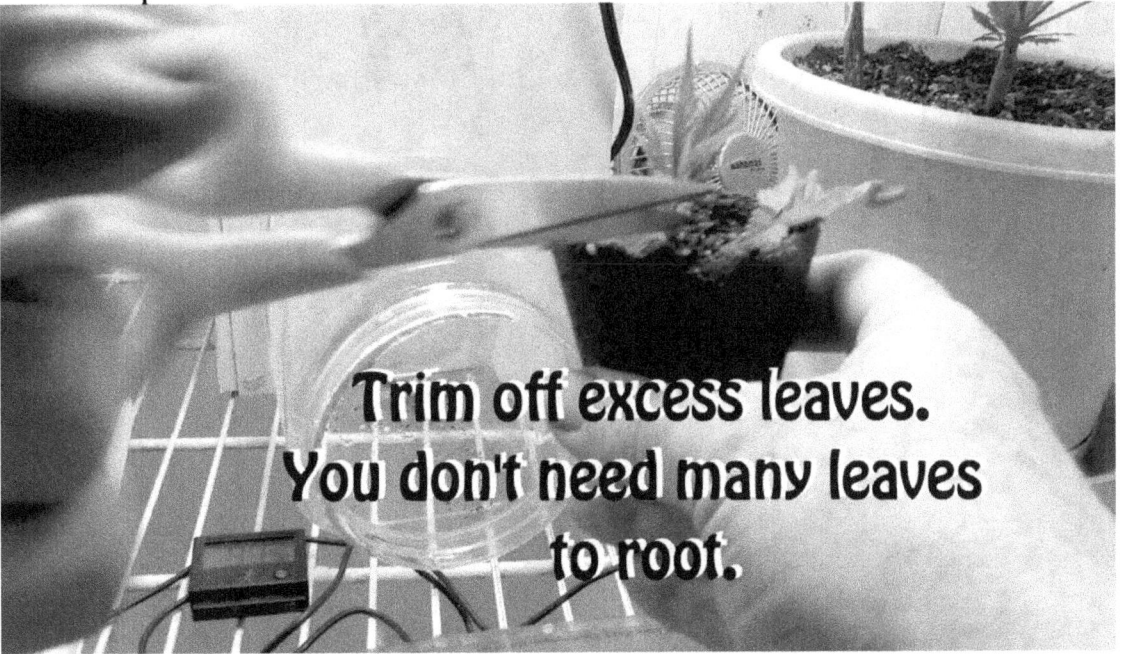

It requires very few leaves or very little leaf area for clones to develop roots, In fact, they can do better with less leaf area as there is less water loss to worry about. Many people cut the leaves in half. (These always eventually die.) and leave only the smallest leaves to root the plant.

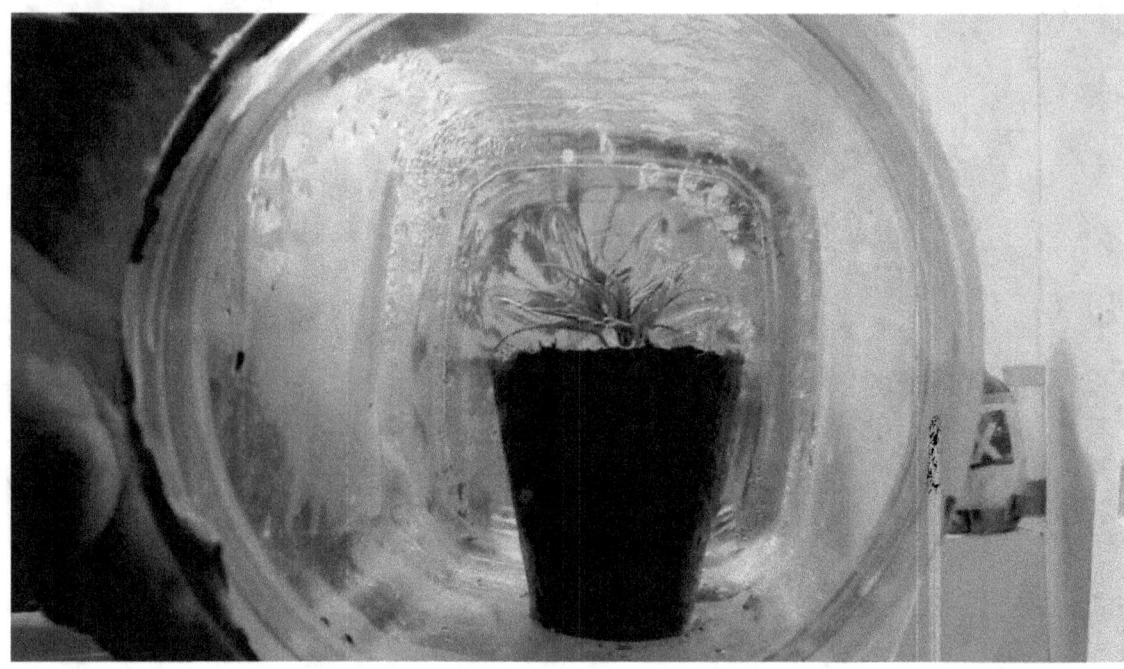

I have used simple jars as a humidity dome, and I have also used commercial domes.   Both work well. The bigger ones do take up a bit of room but usually come with vents that make it easier to lower humidity as time goes by.

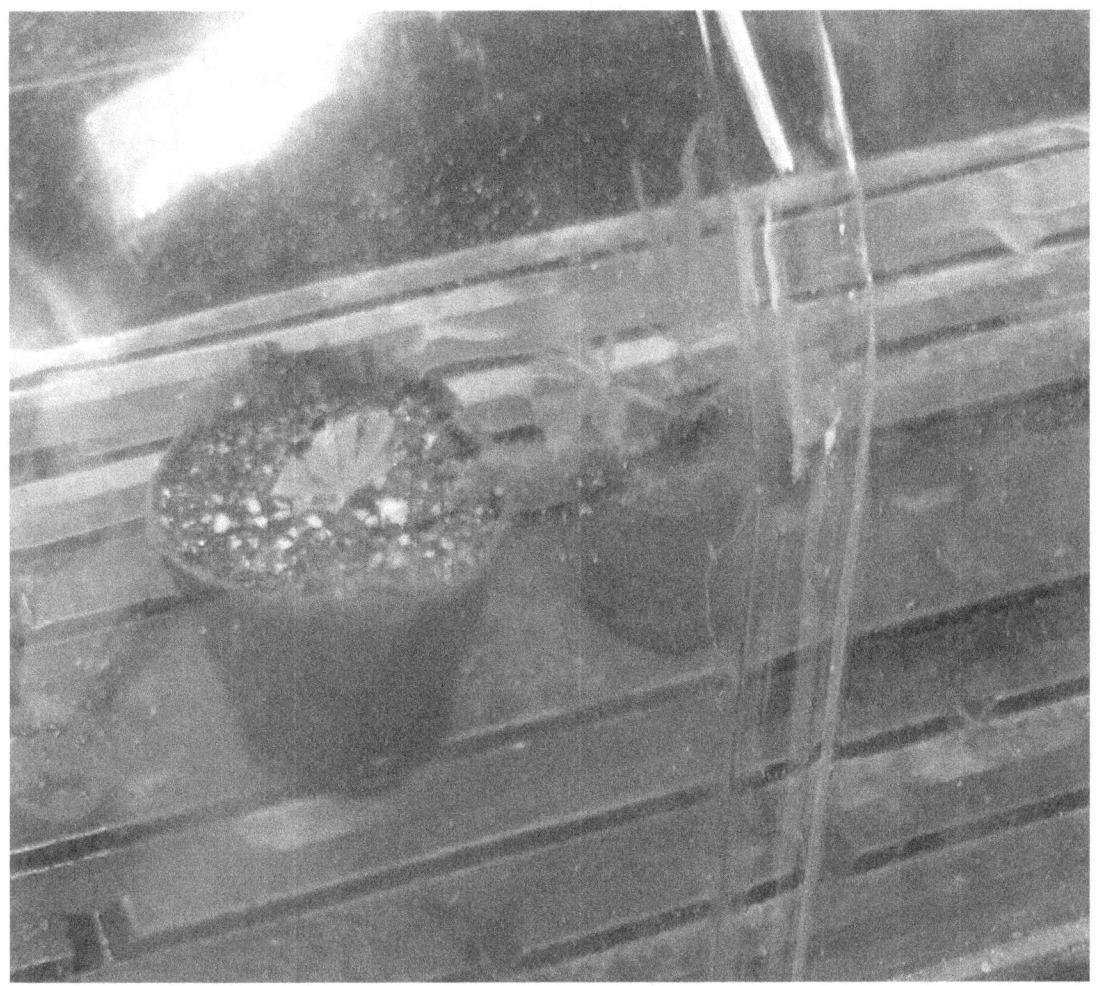

You might find yourself in the situation where you'll need to transport a clone. A pretty good, portable, humidity dome can be made from two soda bottles. Cut so that they fit together. Air holes can be drilled in the sides such that when they line up they let in needed air.

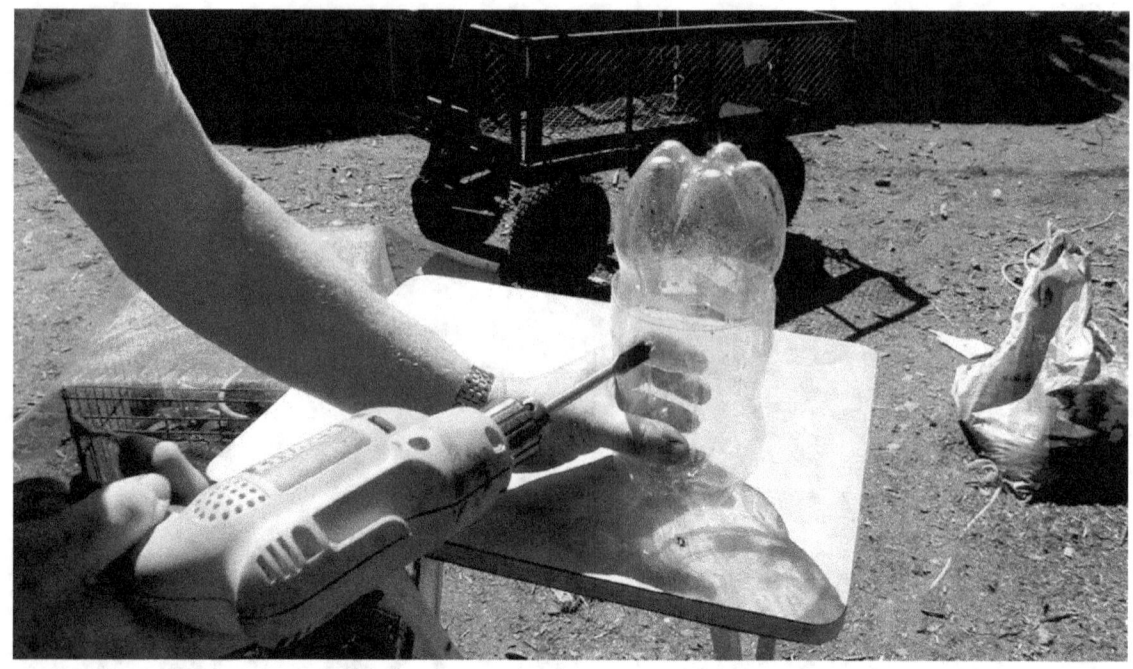

To transport a plant put it in a coir or peat pot that just fits inside the portable dome and secure the pot in place so that it does not bounce around with bubble wrap.

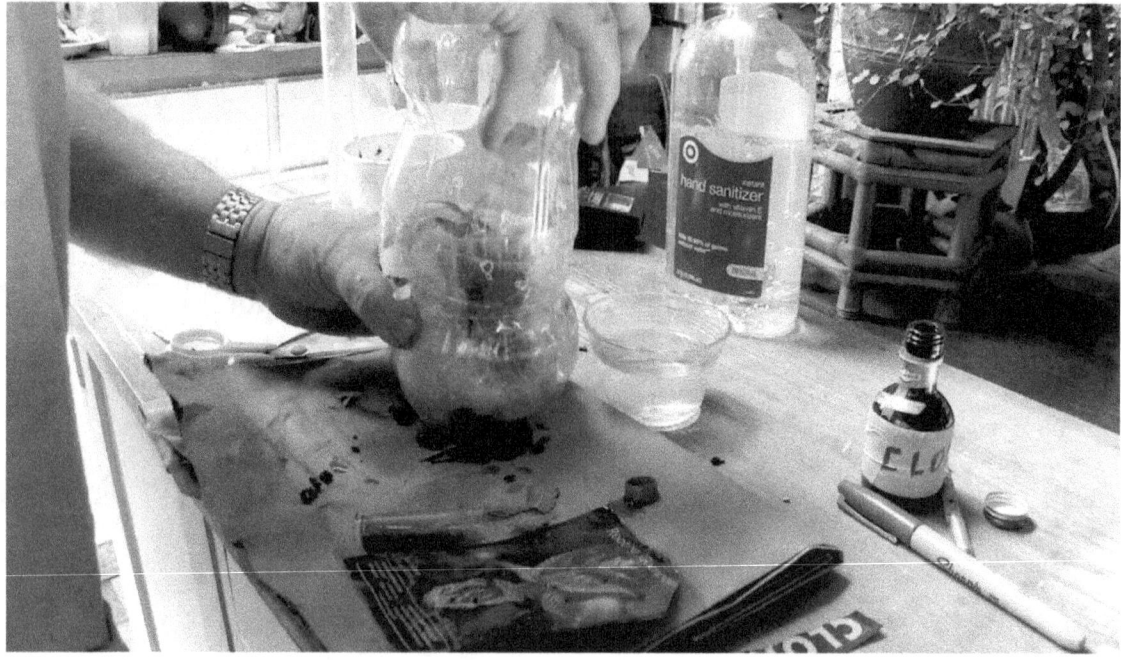

The dome I show above worked very well until I decided to cut a hole in the side to make spraying with nitrosyme solution easier. Even though I covered the hole with duct tape the dome lost humidity and could not be used.

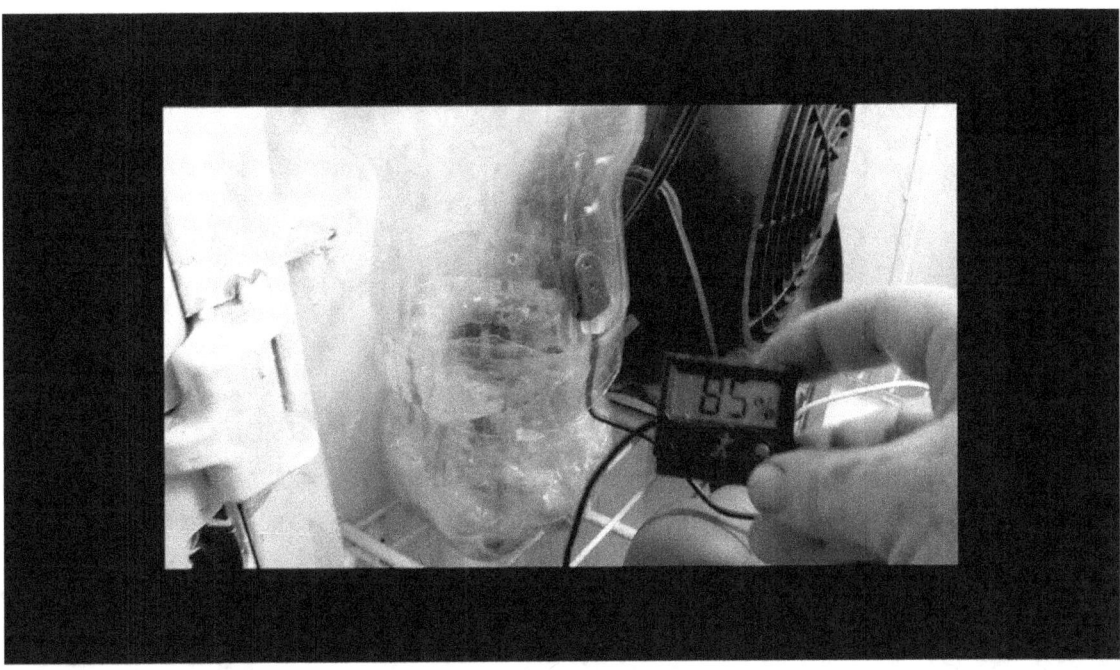

Before I cut a bigger hole in the side the dome easily kept the humidity from 85% to 99%.

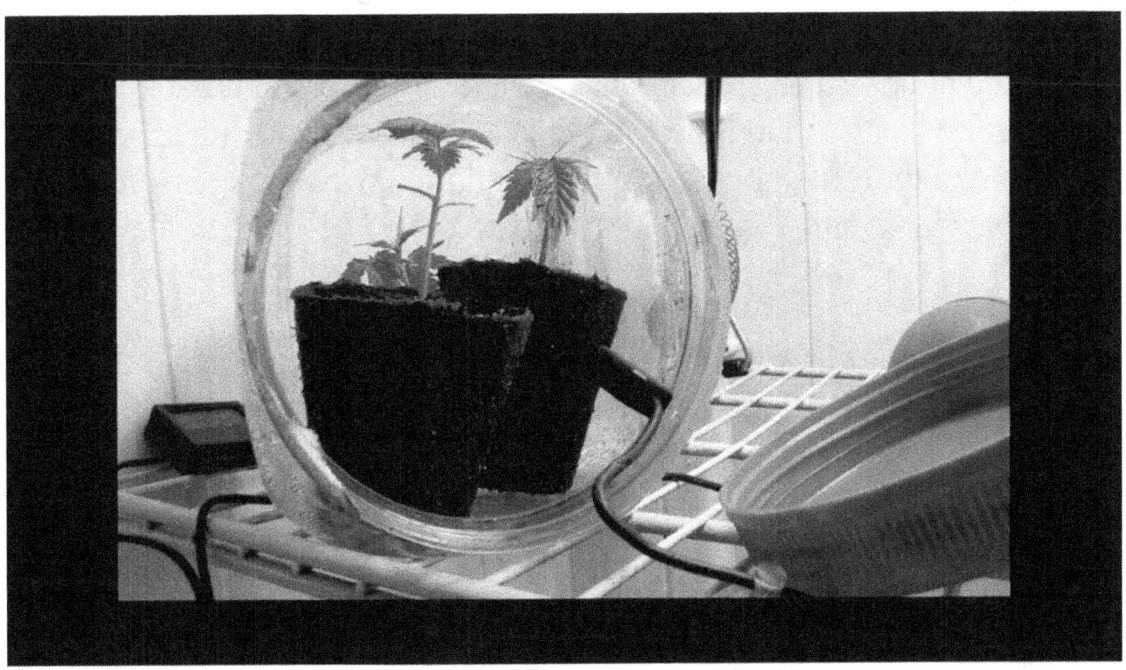

Jars with plants in them will probably stay around 99% humidity if they are sealed. Do let air in every day and spray the leaves with nitrosyme solution.

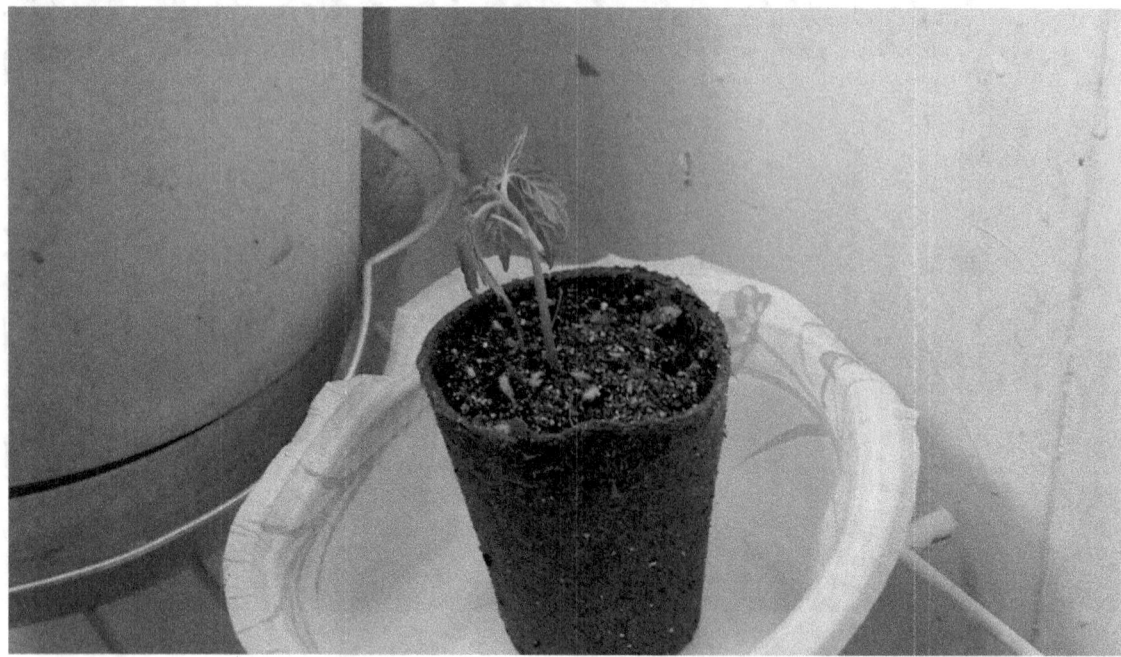

After two weeks you can try taking a clone out, if you've been keeping it in a jar. Or, if you have a dome, try gradually reducing the humidity. Clones are very resilient.[IV] This clone was taken out and began wilting within the hour. Putting it back inside the dome brought it back to life within a few hours. Don't leave a clone just taken from a humidity dome alone for too long. If it does wilt and the root hairs dry out, they may never recover.

[IV] My Iced Grapefruit and Church were reslient when I cloned using Clonex. When I tried a powder cloning agent none of the clones survived.

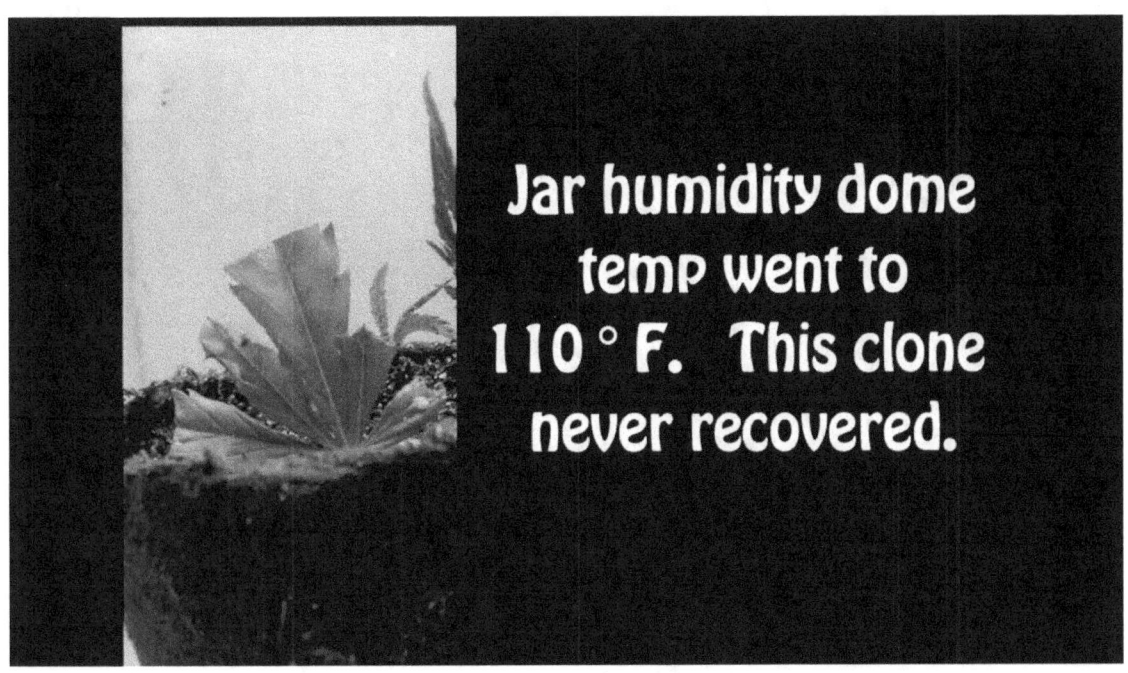

Jar humidity dome temp went to 110° F. This clone never recovered.

Never let a clone get too hot. The one above did when I put it out in the sun. Soil temp went to 110° F. The plant did not die right away but never recovered. If a clone gets to hot start another clone.

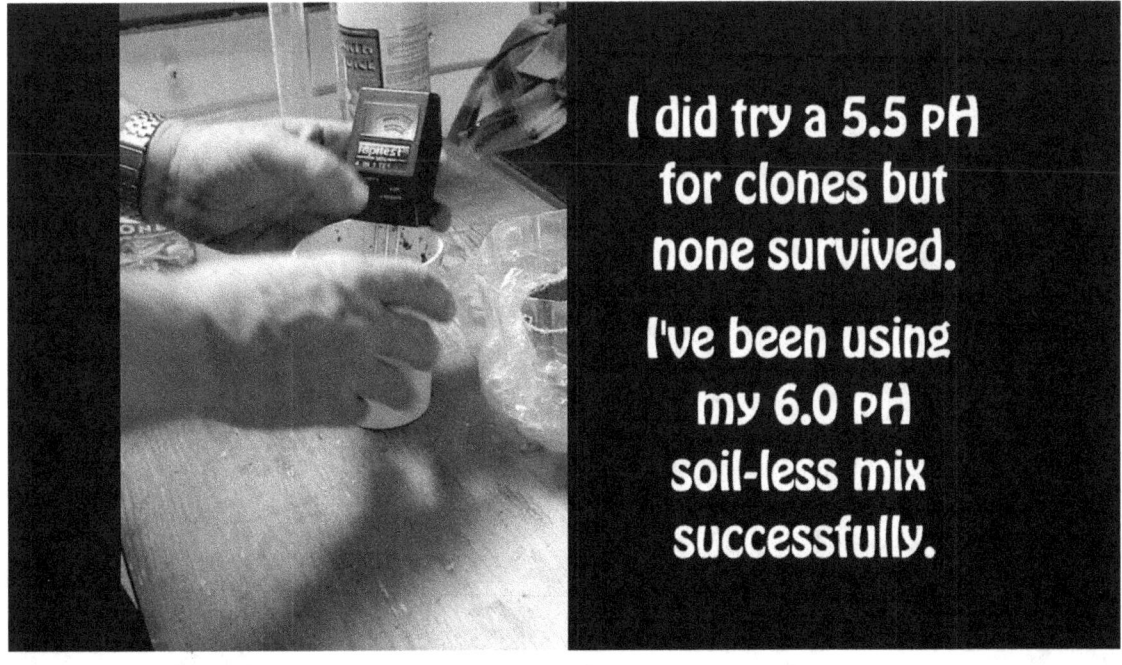

I did try a 5.5 pH for clones but none survived.

I've been using my 6.0 pH soil-less mix successfully.

I have tried lowering the pH of my clones soil-less mix to 5.5 but none survived. So I have been keeping the soil and 6.0 and that has been successful.

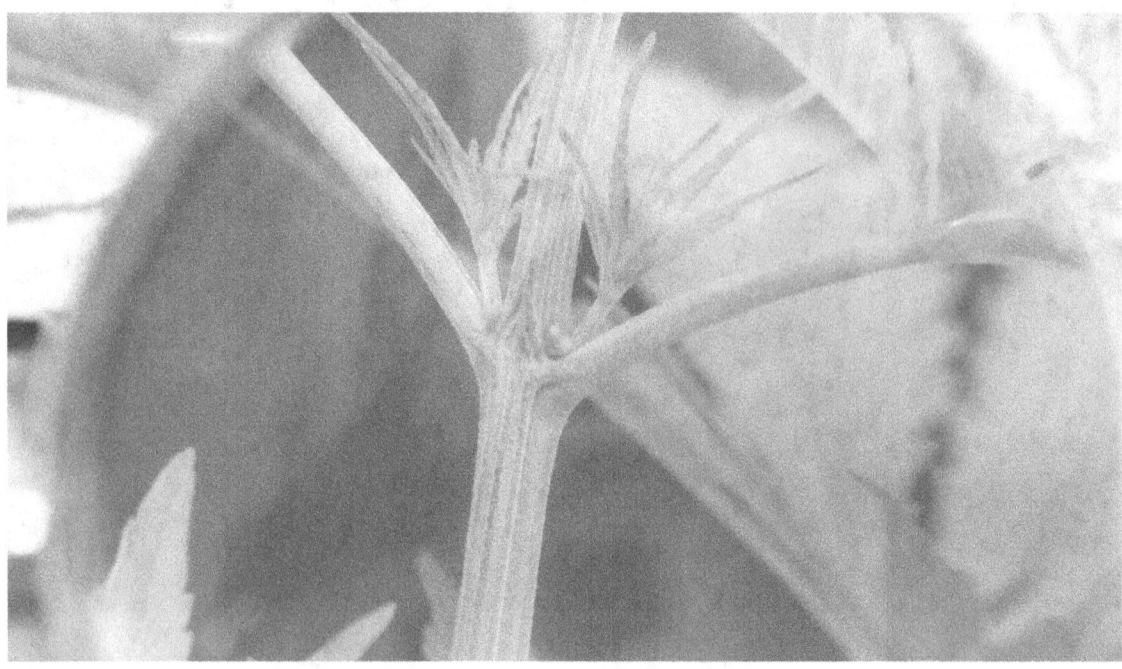

The plant above is a male. It was, unfortunately, the first plant I had that grew. I actually cloned this plant before it showed signs of sexual maturity. Then to my horror I discovered the tiny little multiple bumps or nodes that indicate a male plant.

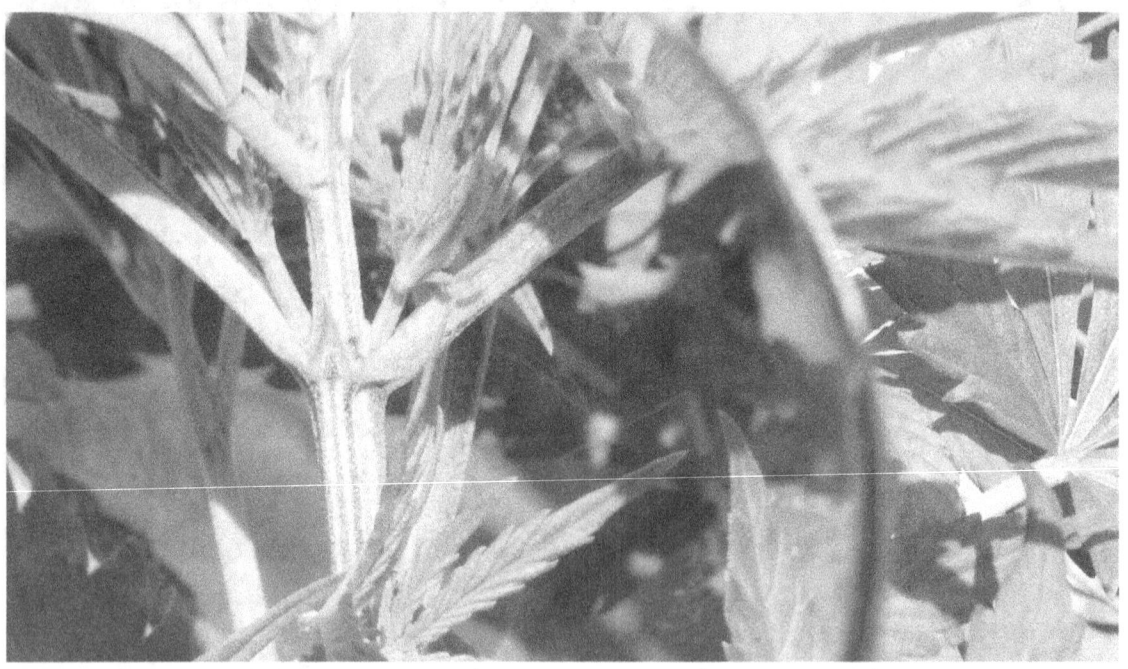

Females have one pear-shaped node, with hairs (pistils) emerging.

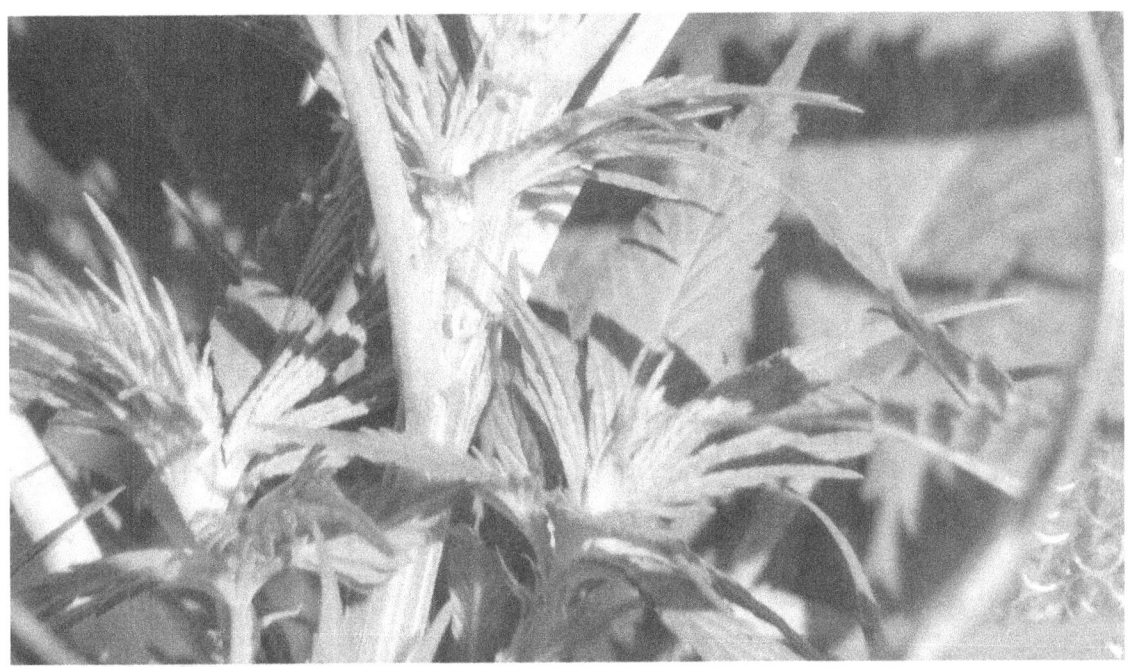

If you do discover you have a male plant you can make of butter[v] out of it, but do not keep it with your female plants, as fertilized females do not produce as much medicine as unfertilized females.

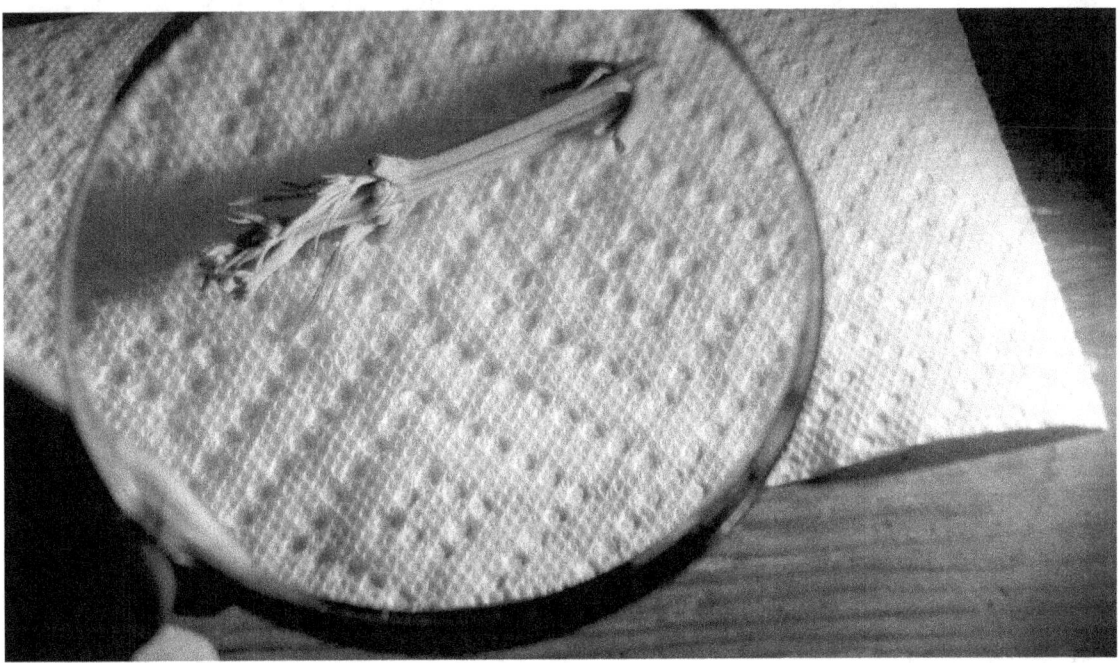

---

[v] Recipies abound on youtube. I also show how to make butter in my much more extensive Learn To Grow Medical Marijuana DVD

You can see the multiple nodes here on this male plant I cut up to make butter with. Even male plants have medicinal qualities. They can be used for tincture or butter. Some people even make hashish out of them but that involves a lot of work and may not be legal in your state. Check out the legality of hash before making it.

Whether you are growing clones or seedlings the moisture content of your soil-less mix is important. The fast-draining soil-less mix designed here will help you plants keep from getting to wet, but they can dry out. Learn to pinch your soil. The unique feel of wet sand in our mix should tell you right away if the pot needs watering.

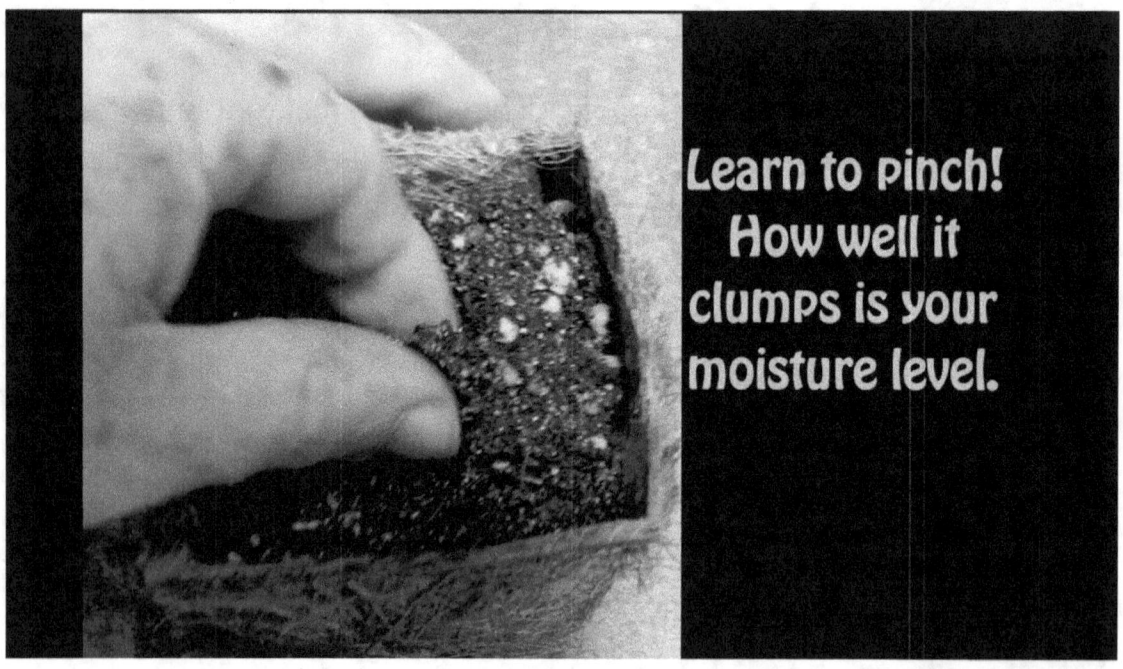

Learn to pinch! How well it clumps is your moisture level.

Your fertilizers are an important part of your medicine growing and you will need some sort of measured flask to mix them. I use a 100 ml graduated cylinder, a 450 ml graduated cylinder and a 25 ml graduated cylinder—using the 25 ml graduated cylinder most often. I also use an eye dropper.

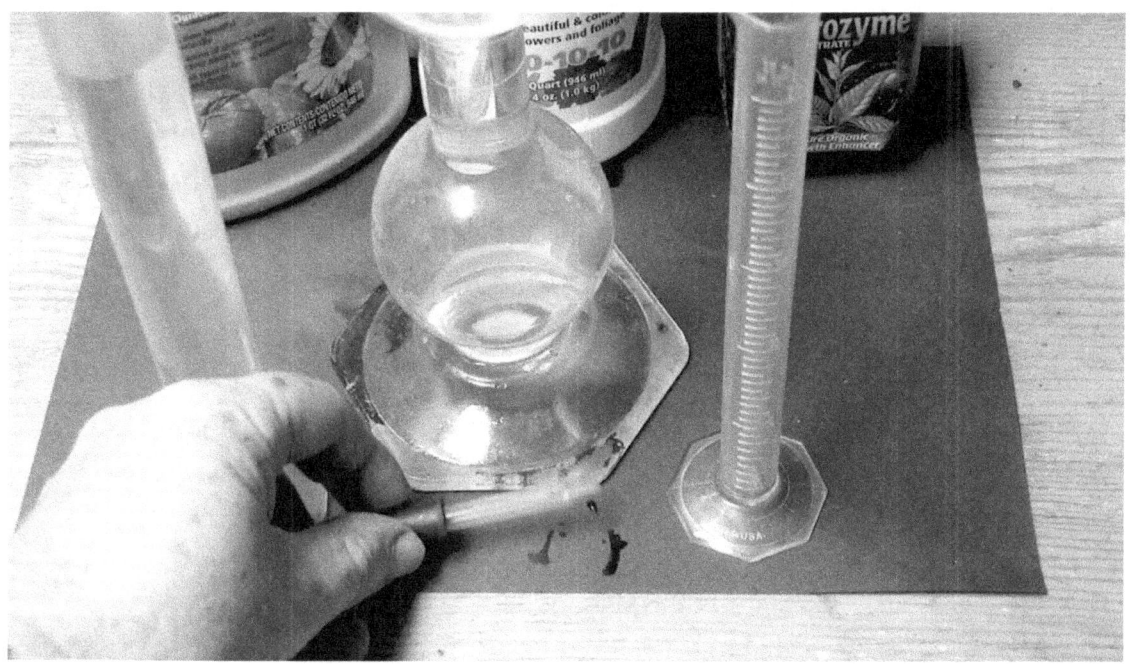

You need to calibrate your eye dropper. I made use of the fact that one ml of distilled water weighs one gram. I weighed out one gram of water droplets and found it took 20 drops to make that gram. Alternatively, you could count how many drops it takes to measure out one ml of water in your graduated cylinder. I don't usually measure out more fertilizer than needed, so often made small amounts, especially when starting out.

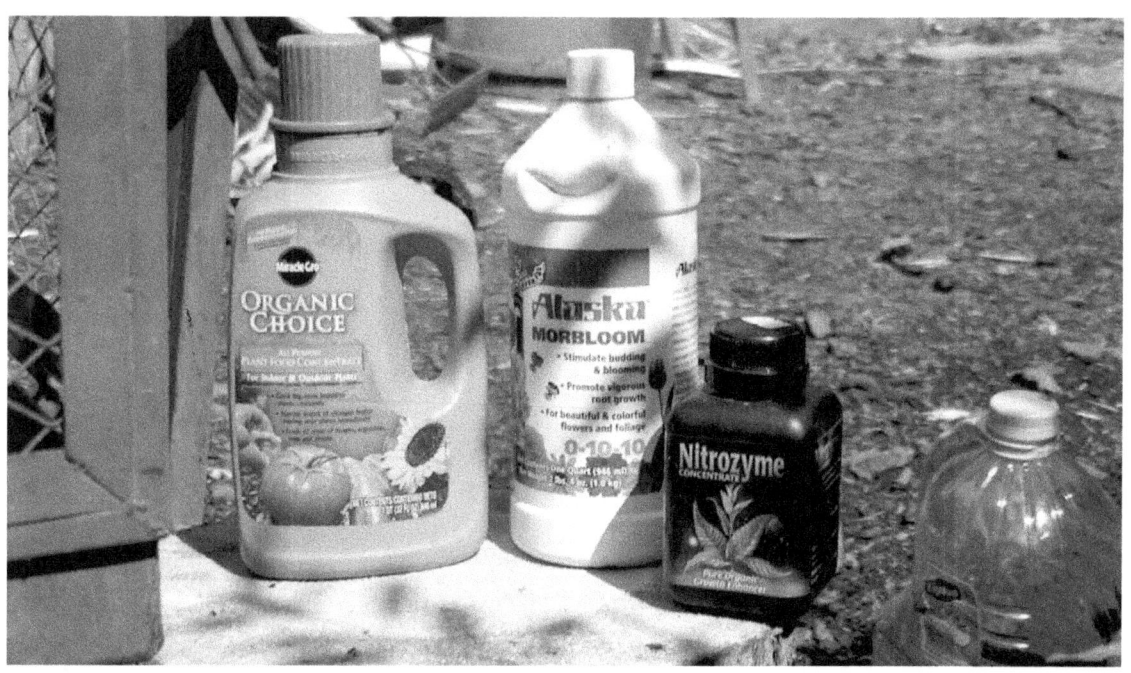

For my fertilizers I chose those I could find at local hardware or garden shops. I chose Miracle Grow Organic Choice as my fertilizer and Alaska MoreBloom 0-10-10 as my bloom fertilizer. I added nitrosyme (or Liquid Seaweed) to all fertilizer solutions as well as making up a .5% nitrosyme solution for foliar feeding.

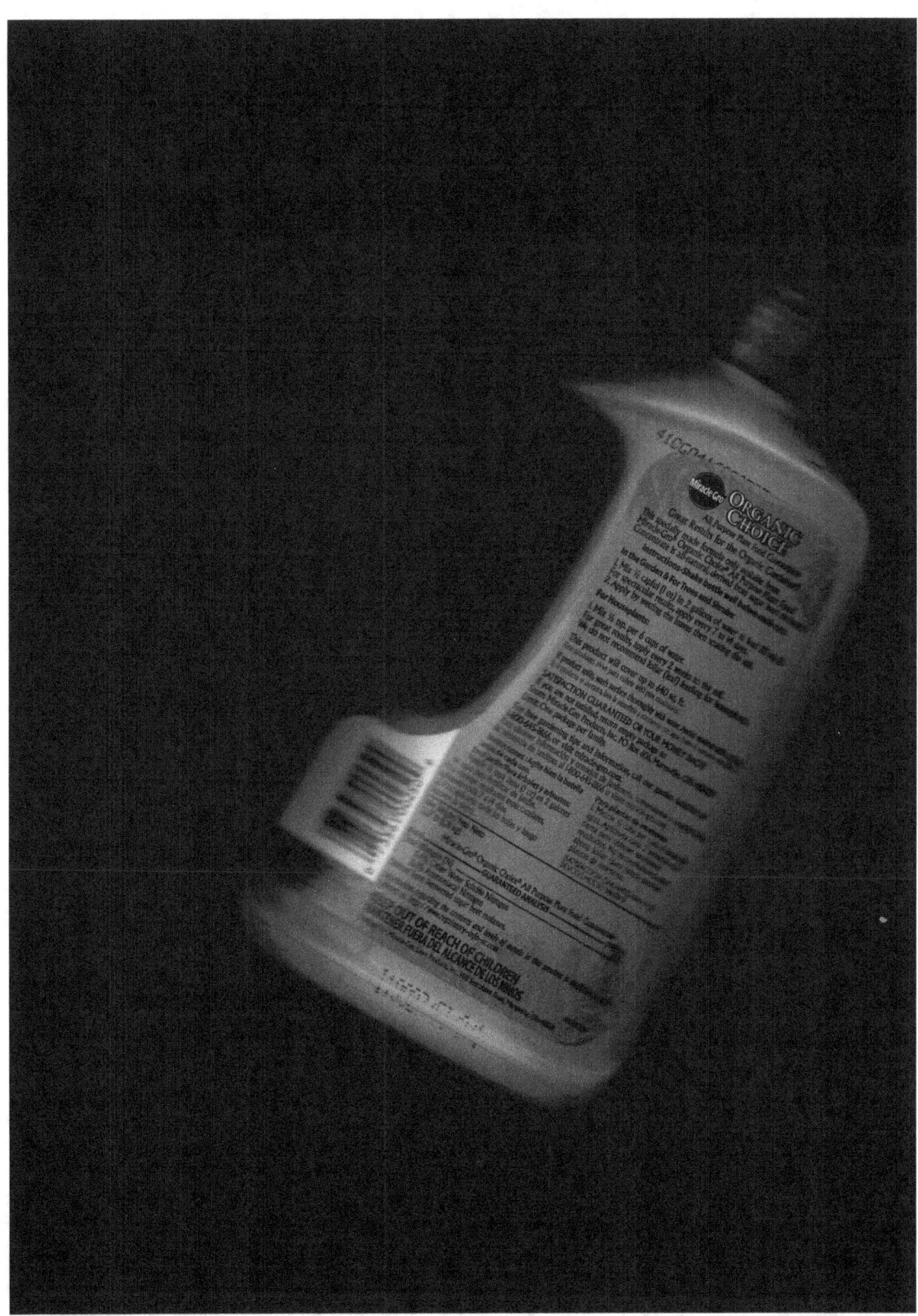

Instructions for using fertilizer can be found on the back of the fertilizer bottle. I choose the formula on this bottle for houseplants. Then I made a ¼ Strength mix.

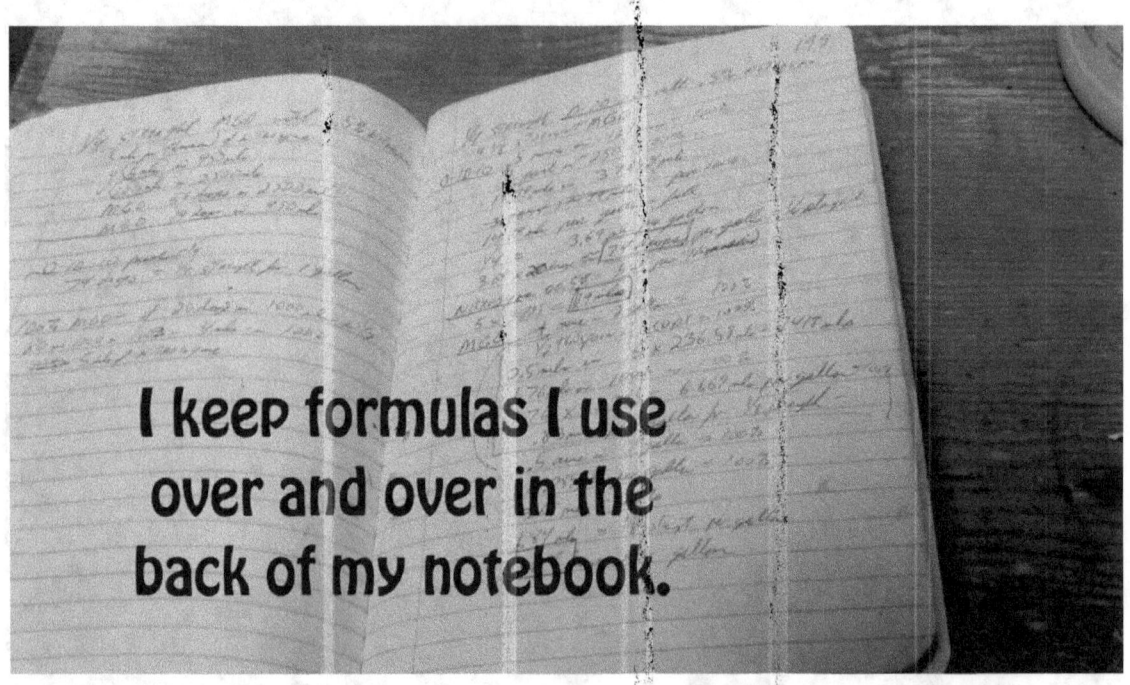

I keep formulas I use over and over in the back of my notebook.

I tend to be heavy handed with my watering. This can be a problem as too much fertilizer can burn your leaf tips. By using ¼ strength solution I can be heavy handed and the plants won't suffer all that much. At the first sign of leaf tip damage I just switch to plain water for awhile.

Underwatering
Overwatering
Underfertilization
Overfertilization

pH to High
pH to Low

A
Lack
Of
Oxygen

In fact, by using my soil-less mix and a `1/4 strength fertilizer solution we can narrow down the problems we are likely to see in our growing.

Our soil-less mix makes over-watering less likely. It is not impossible to over-water. If you constantly saturated the soil it could get wet enough to cause rotting problems, but with normal watering this is unlikely. And if the plants do get too much water all you have to do is let the pot dry out a bit.

Under-watering can be a real problem. Don't let your plants dry out as dried out rootlets will not recover.

Our plants' roots need oxygen to grow. This is one of the reasons we use perlite (below) in our mix. The faceted surface of this mineral traps air molecules that that roots can get to.

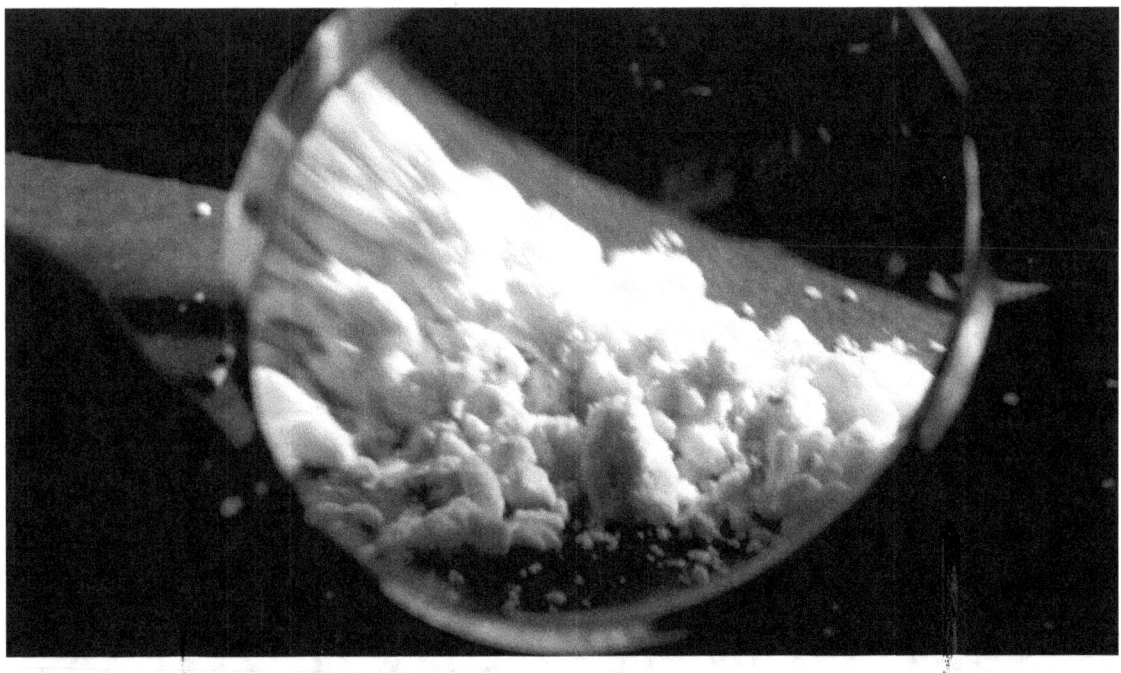

By using perlite and always shaking our fertilizer solutions and/or water before watering or fertilizing will guarantee our plant roots always have the necessary oxygen.

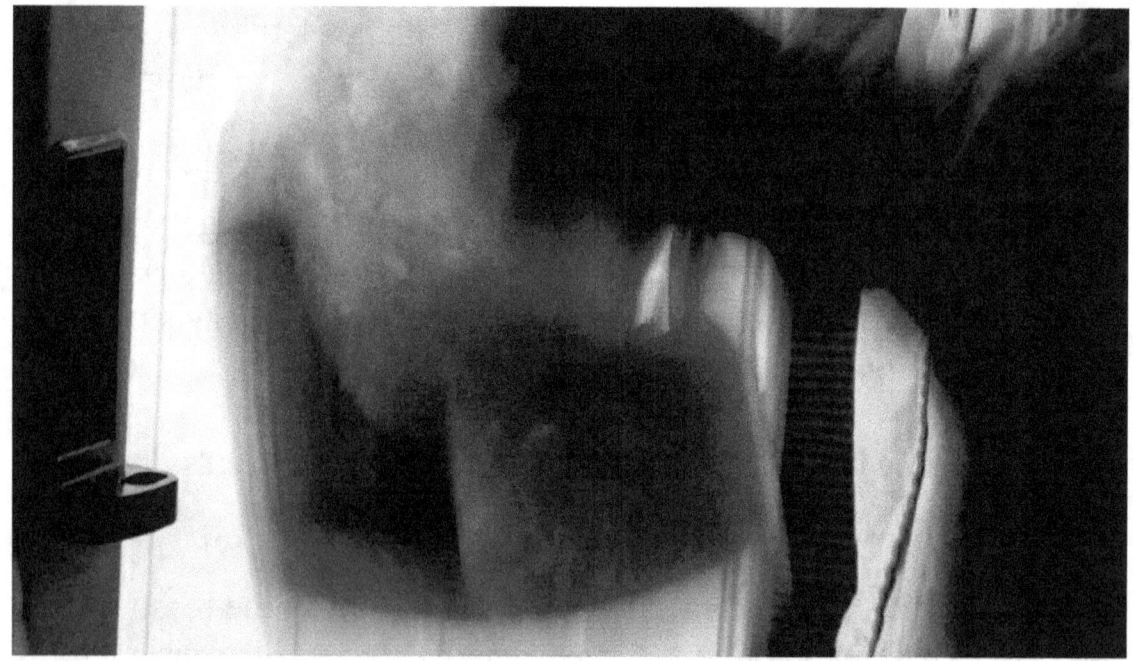

I try to use unique bottles for each solution. The one pictured above contains my bloom fertilizer. Vigorously shaking will make the solution froth and this means there will be plenty of oxygen for our roots.

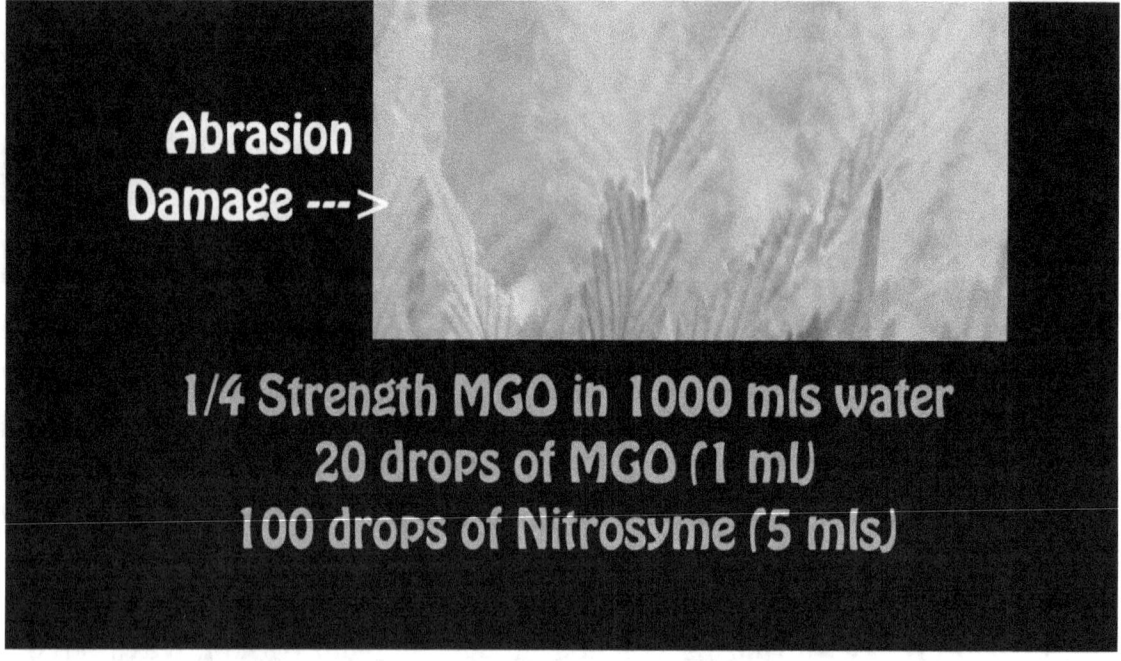

Abrasion
Damage --->

1/4 Strength MGO in 1000 mls water
20 drops of MGO (1 ml)
100 drops of Nitrosyme (5 mls)

To make sure I don't over-fertilize, I use, as mentioned earlier, a ¼ strength solution of my fertilizers.

You'll note in the seedling photo below its leaf tip shows some discoloration. This is from over-fertilization. Actually, seedlings should not be fertilized at all until they are at least 21 days old. This seedling was over-fertilized because it was fertilized too early.

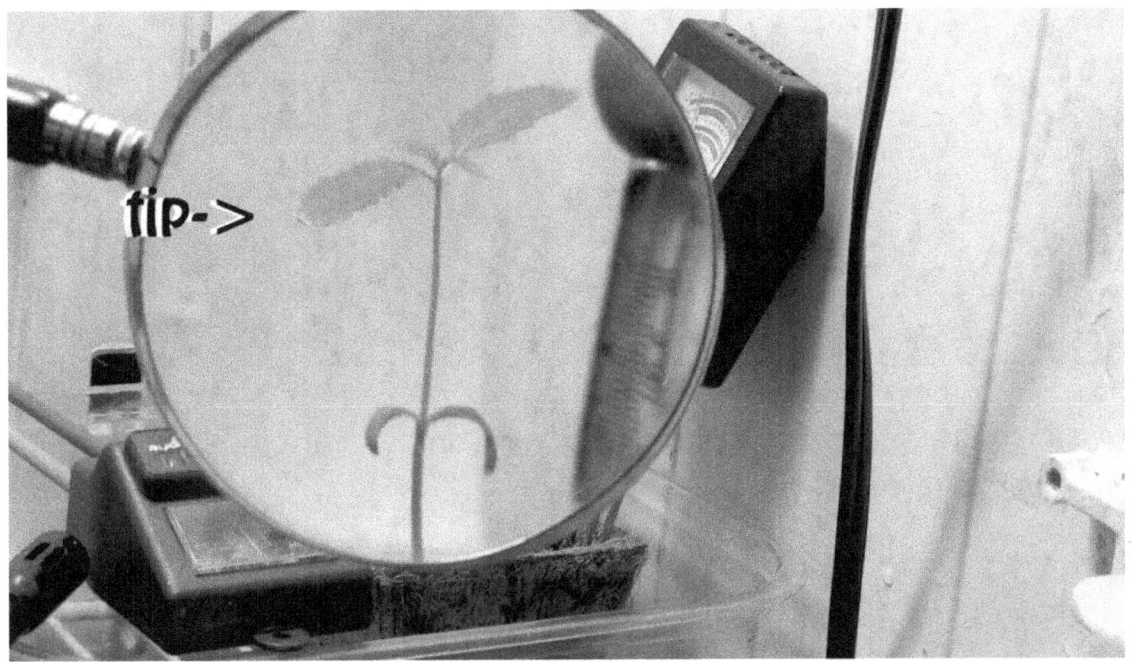

As an over-fertilized plant grows the leaf tip damage moves down the plant.

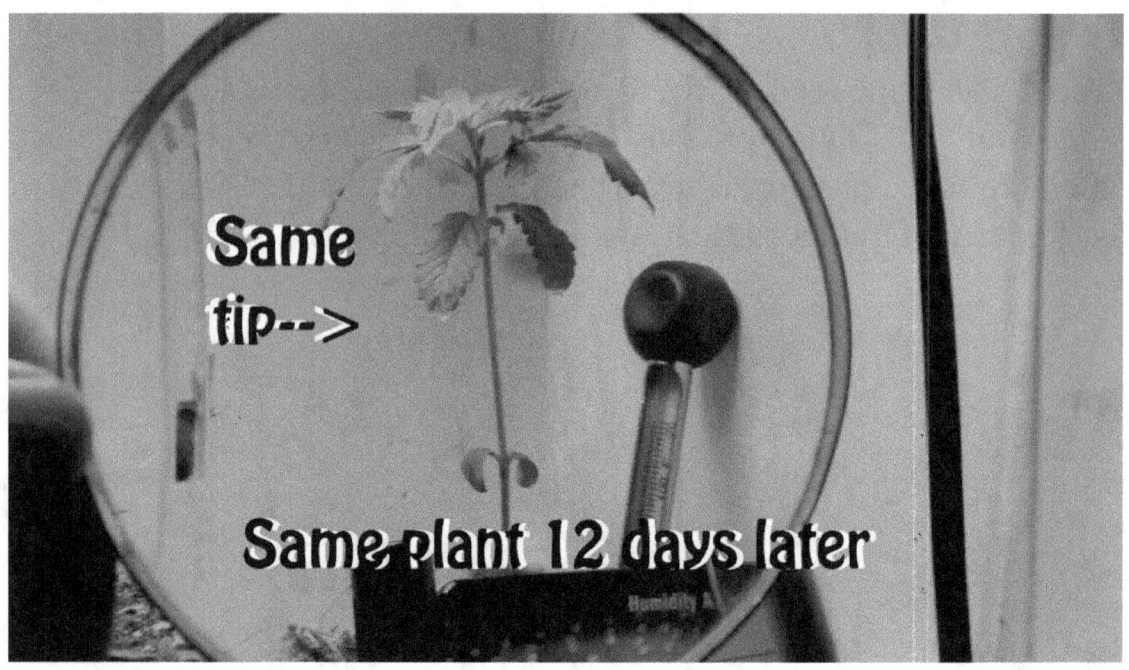

Again, if you see signs of over-fertilization and you are using a ¼ strength solution, all you have to do is:

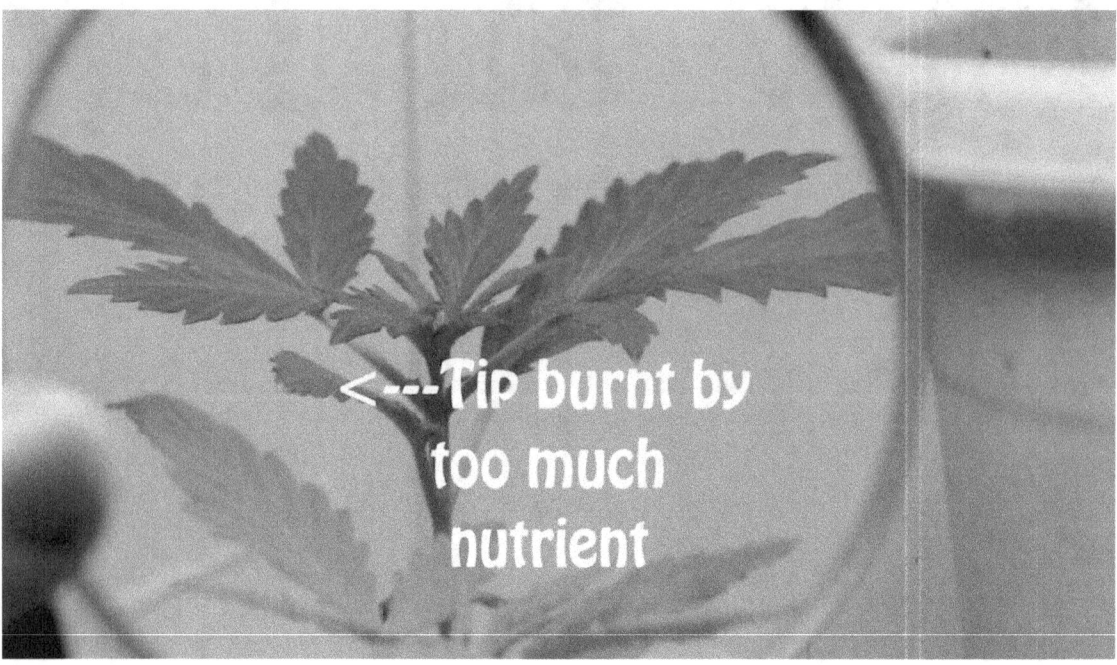

Identify the leaf tip damage.

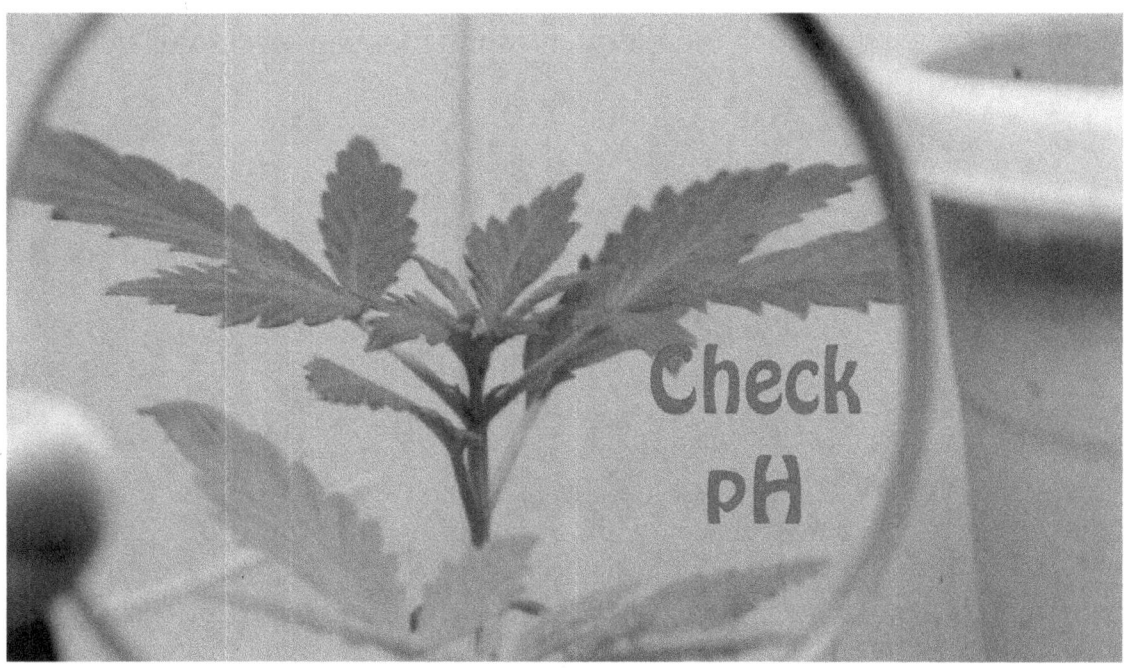

Check the soil pH. If he soil is not 6.0 then adjust and wait a day or so to see what happens. If the damage continues flush your soil-less mix with water to remove the excess fertilizer.

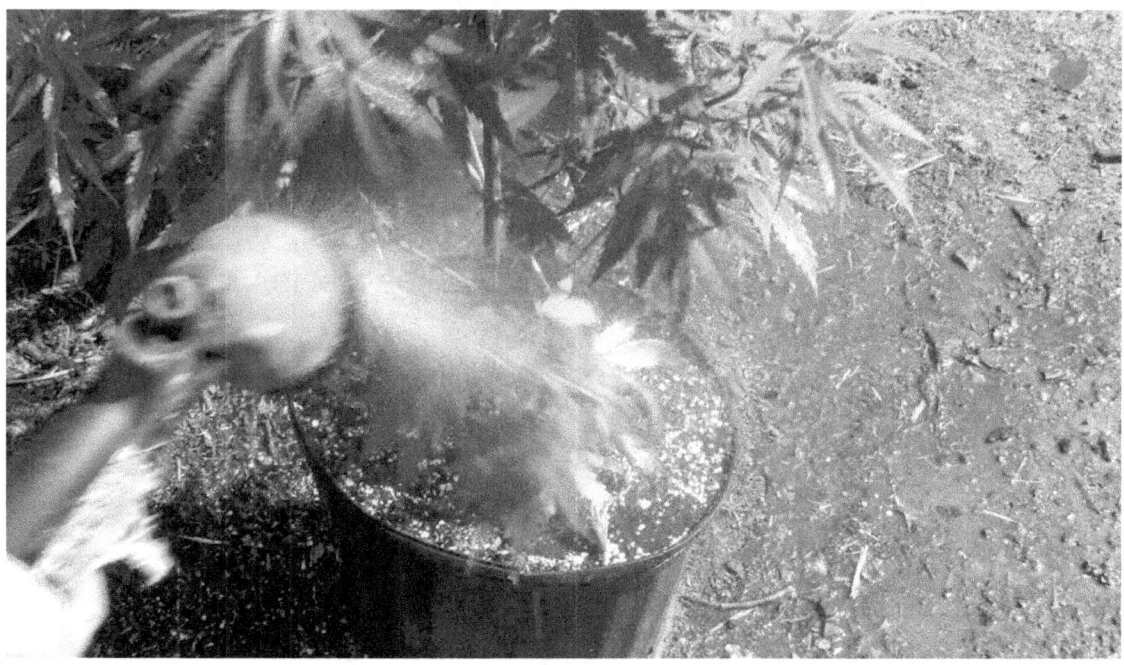

Flushing can remove not only excess fertilizer but fertilizer salt buildup (Products of fertilizer use by the plant). In fact, before moving a plant from the growing shed to the blooming shed many growers flush the soil with water.

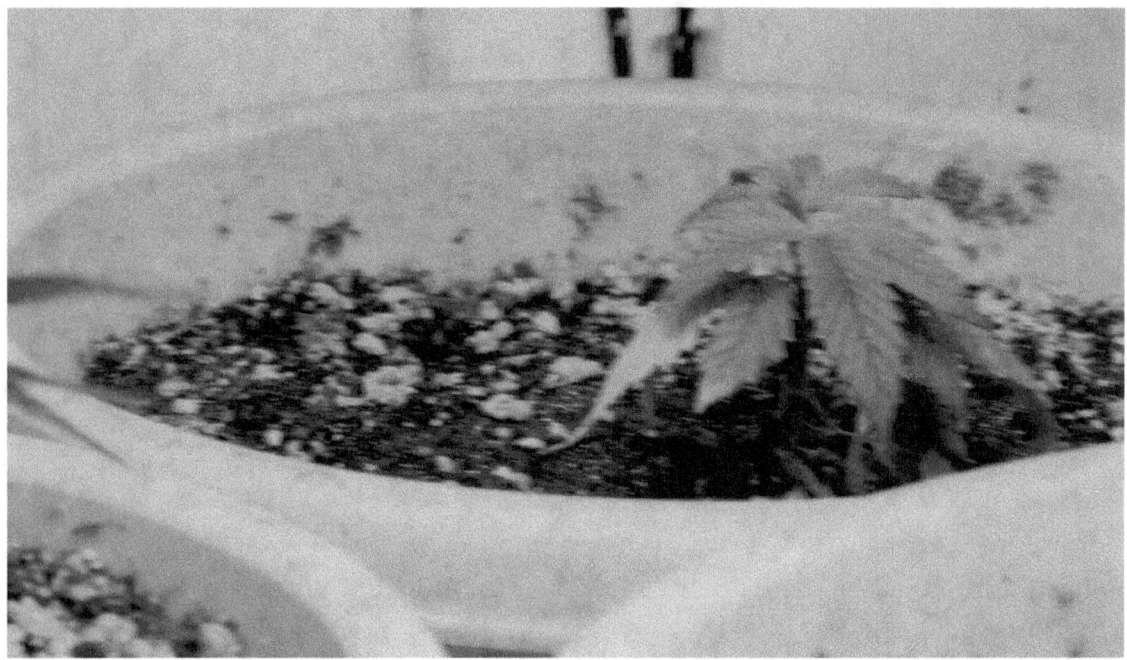

Under-fertilization can also occur, although it is usually more plant specific. Above a Bubba Kush[VI] plant is showing yellow leaves. This indicates under-fertilization.

I tried fertilizing more often with my ¼ strength fertilizer but the leaves stayed yellow. When I mixed up a 100% mixture of MGO the yellow went away and the plant began growing as shown below.

[VI] I found Bubba Kush very difficult to bloom and more difficult to clone and don't recommend it for my LED system.

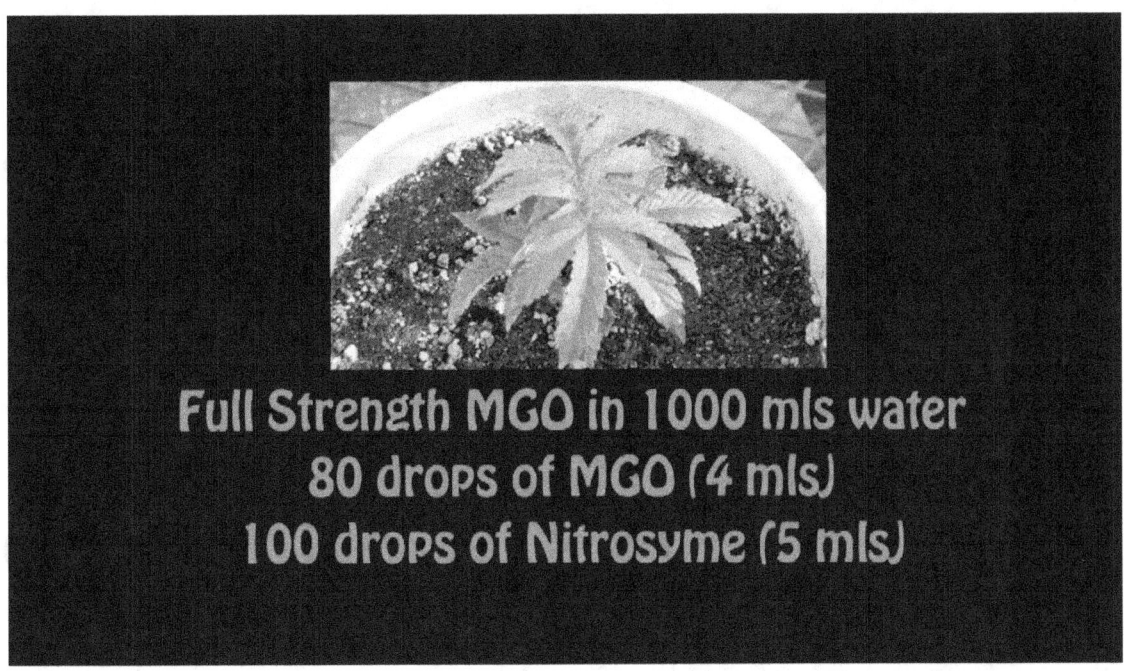

Full Strength MGO in 1000 mls water
80 drops of MGO (4 mls)
100 drops of Nitrosyme (5 mls)

Under-fertilization, however, isn't the only reason a plant might yellow. Fertilizers other than ones intended for foliar use can burn a plant if splash on the leaves. If you see yellowing check to see if there is a pattern to the yellow area.

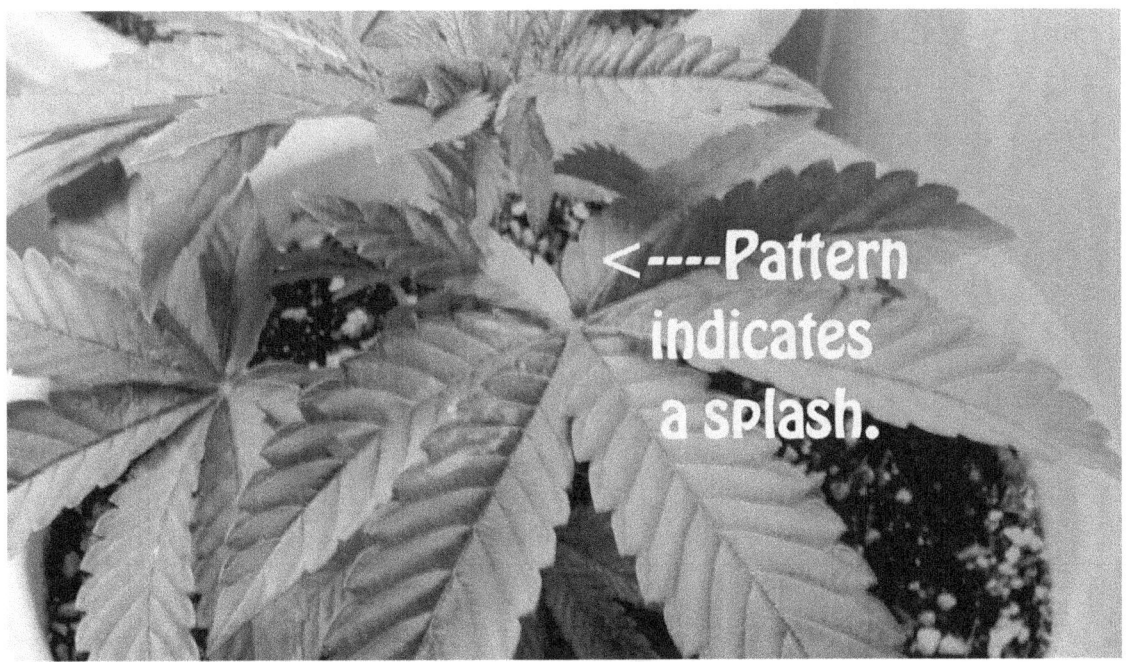

<----Pattern indicates a splash.

The yellow color will look similar to that of a fertilizer deficiency but the splash-like pattern will indicate a splash burn. If you realize you've splashed your plant use some distilled water in a mister and mist the splashed fertilizer off.

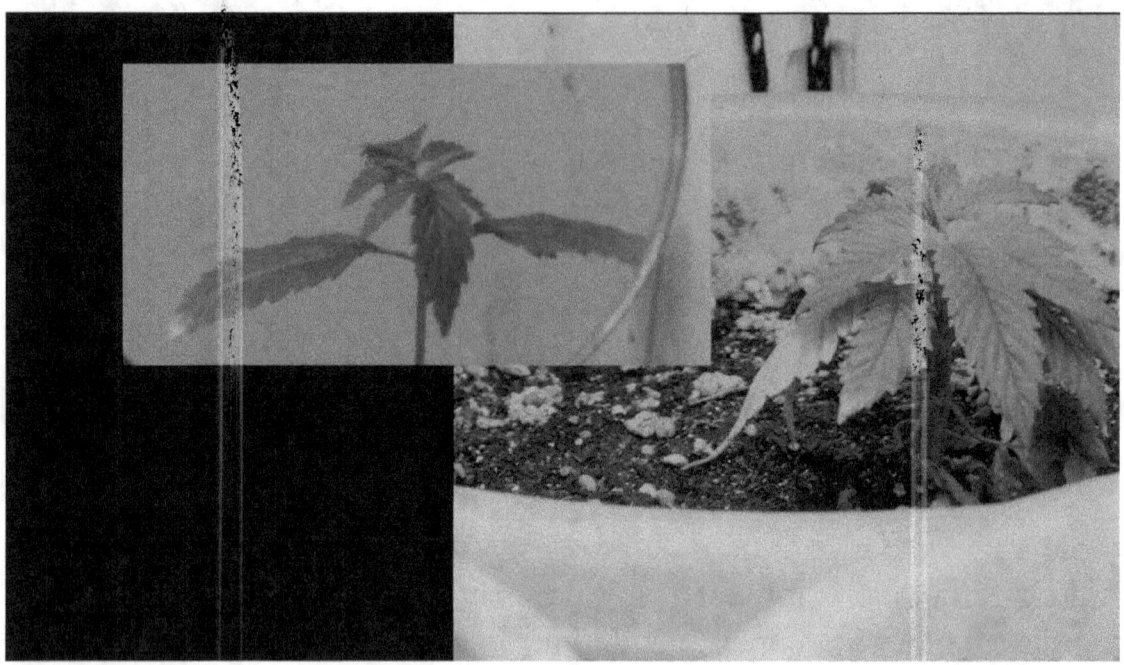

The main reason I choose my soil-less mix and ¼ strength fertilizer solution is that only two problems are likely to present themselves. First if you use too much of the ¼ strength solution the tips will burn. Or, the plant will not get enough fertilizer (indicating a plant that needs higher levels of nutrients)..

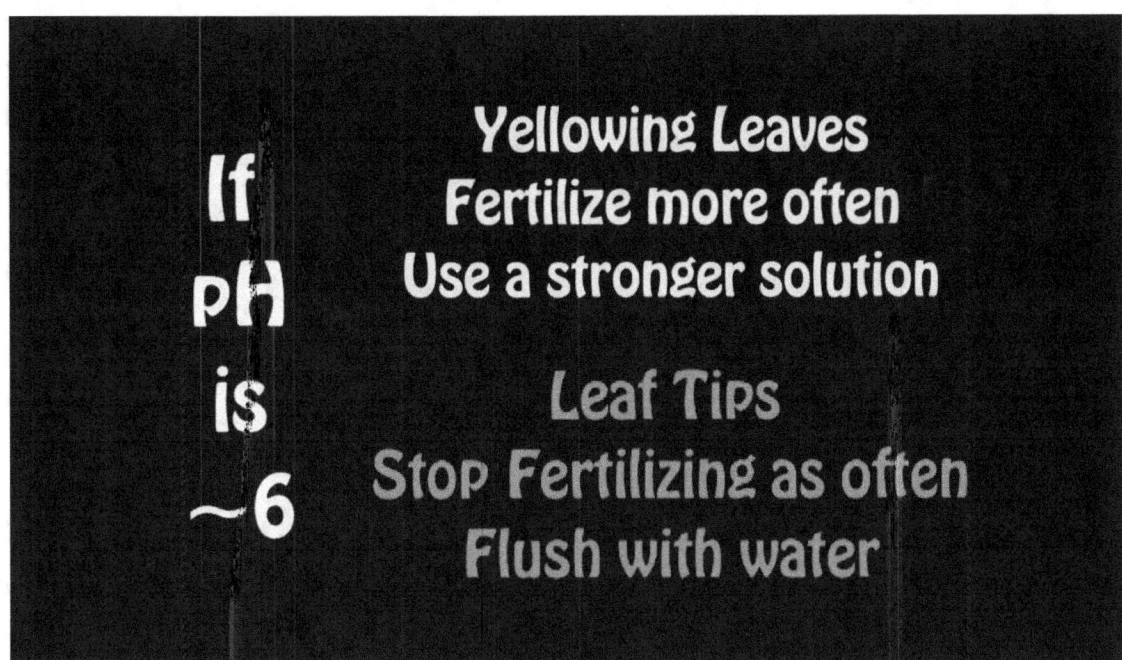

The solution in either case is easy.

First: Make sure the pH is around 6.0.

If the pH is not at 6.0 add natural Down or Natural Up to set the pH in the correct range.

Cut back on the fertilizer if you see tip burn.

If the plant is yellowing, make sure it is not caused by an errant splash of fertilizer. And if the yellowing was not a splash, make up and use a stronger fertilizer solution.

Do check your soil moisture every day. I've mentioned this earlier but it will be a fatal mistake if you make it.

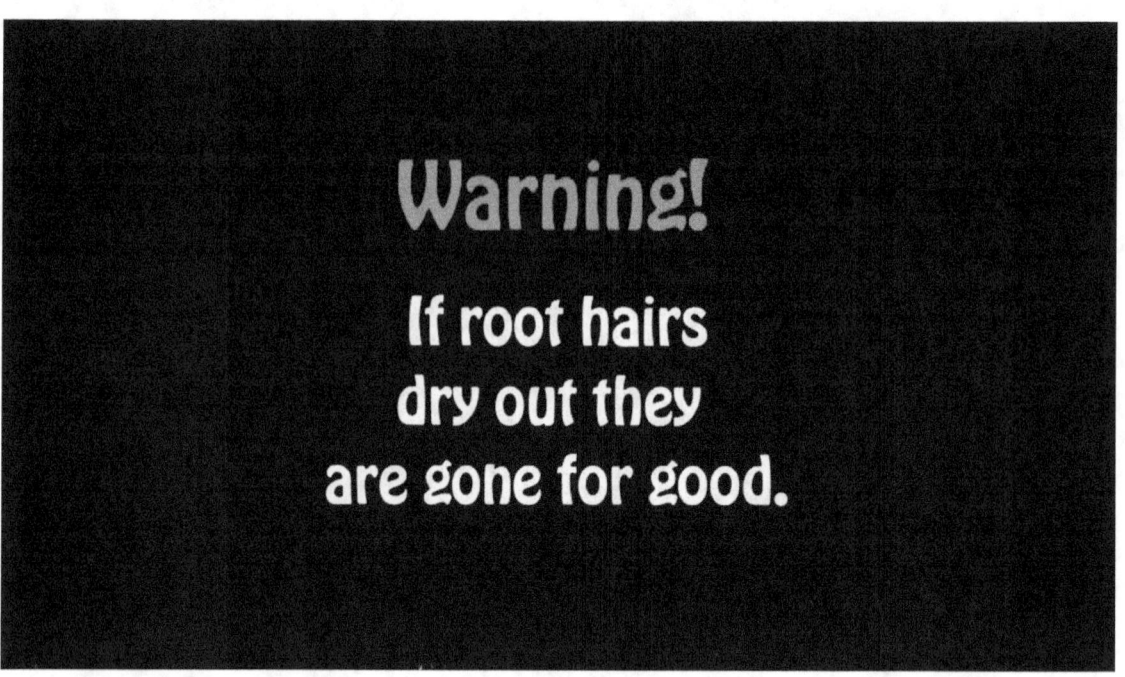

Warning!

**If root hairs
dry out they
are gone for good.**

Over-watering with our fast draining soil is harder to do, but not impossible. The plant below started dropping after it was watered heavily just before lights out for the night. In the morning it was drooping from too much water, but perked up as soon as the grow lights came on and it had a chance to dry a bit.

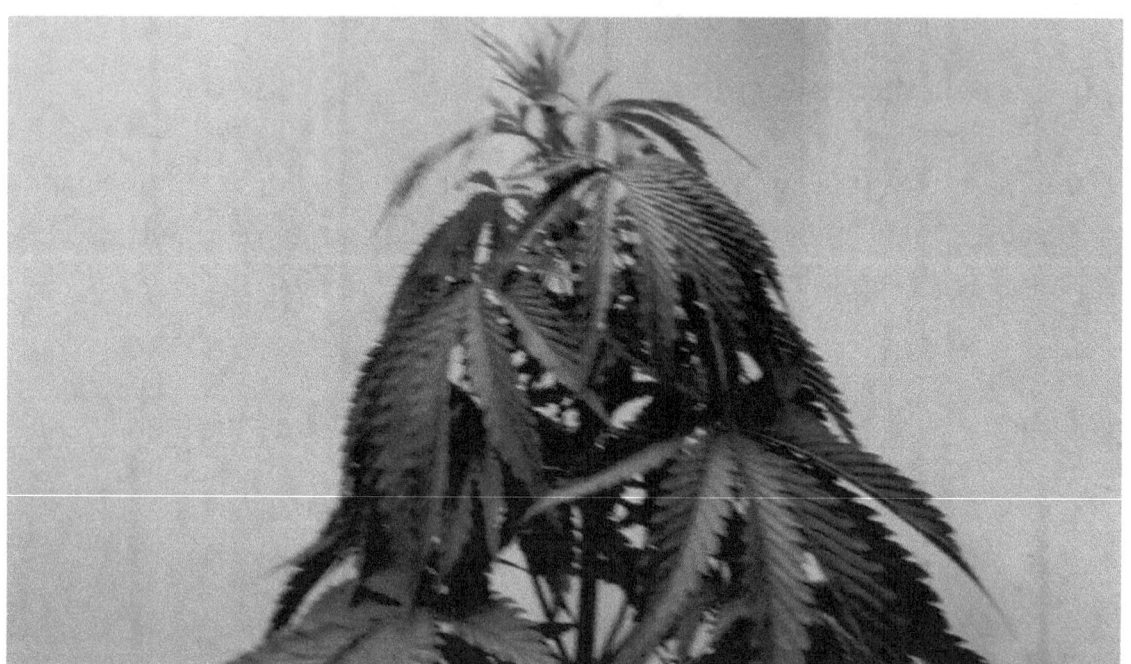

By the way having the right tools always makes things easier. When watering keep a baster on hand to remove excess water.

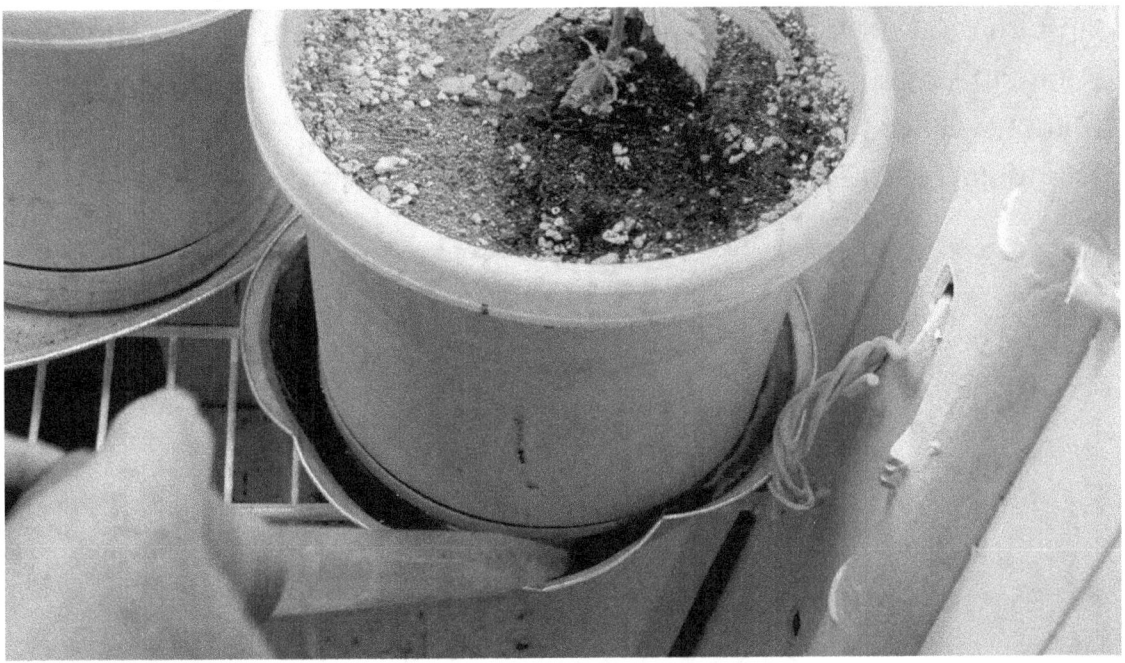

You're going to need pots to grow your plants in. The bigger the pot the less likely you'll run out of water, but then larger pots take up room and we have limited room in our small grow sheds.

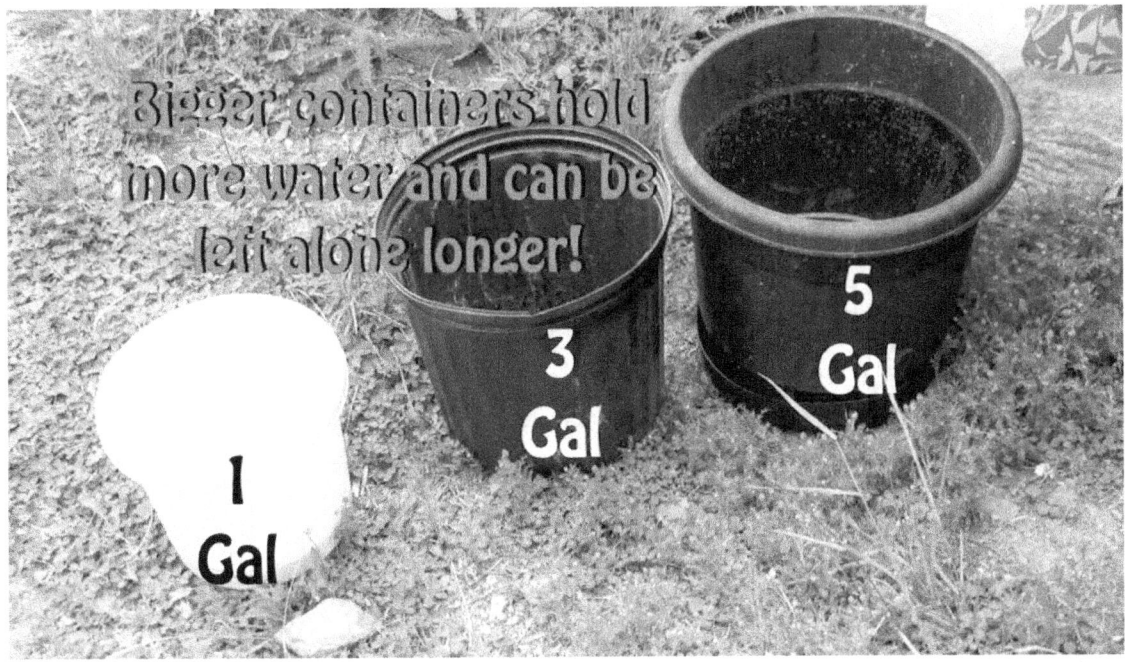

I use one gallon pots in my grow shed. Then transfer my plants to 3 gallon pots when they bloom. The plants will need the extra root room for maximum growth. You might also want to keep a 5 gallon pot on hand if you want to keep a mother plant for cloning. In theory a mother plant can keep growing in the 'grow' stage indefinitely. The growing mother will need a bit more root room. One and three gallon pots will be enough for most of your growing needs.

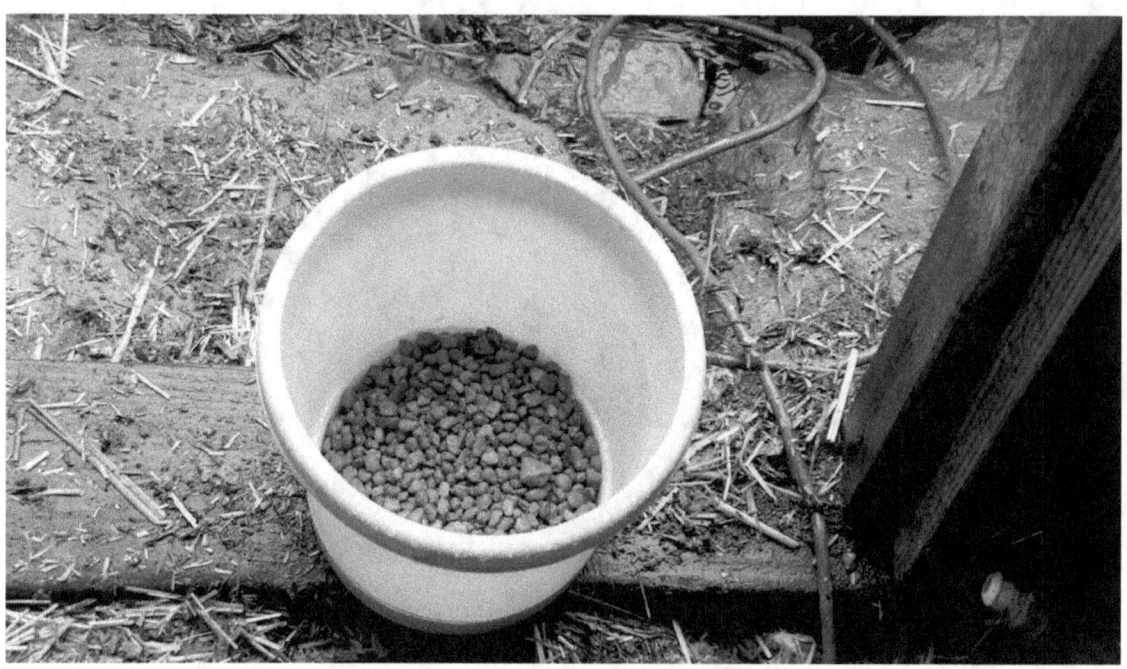

The first repotting you'll be doing is when you take your clone or seedling from it's small pot and move the plant to your one gallon container.

I always fill the bottom of my pots with pebbles for draining. Water will be pool in the pebbles and I always see evidence on harvest or replanting that my plants have extend rootlets into the pebbles for moisture. This is way soil-less is very much like hydroponics.

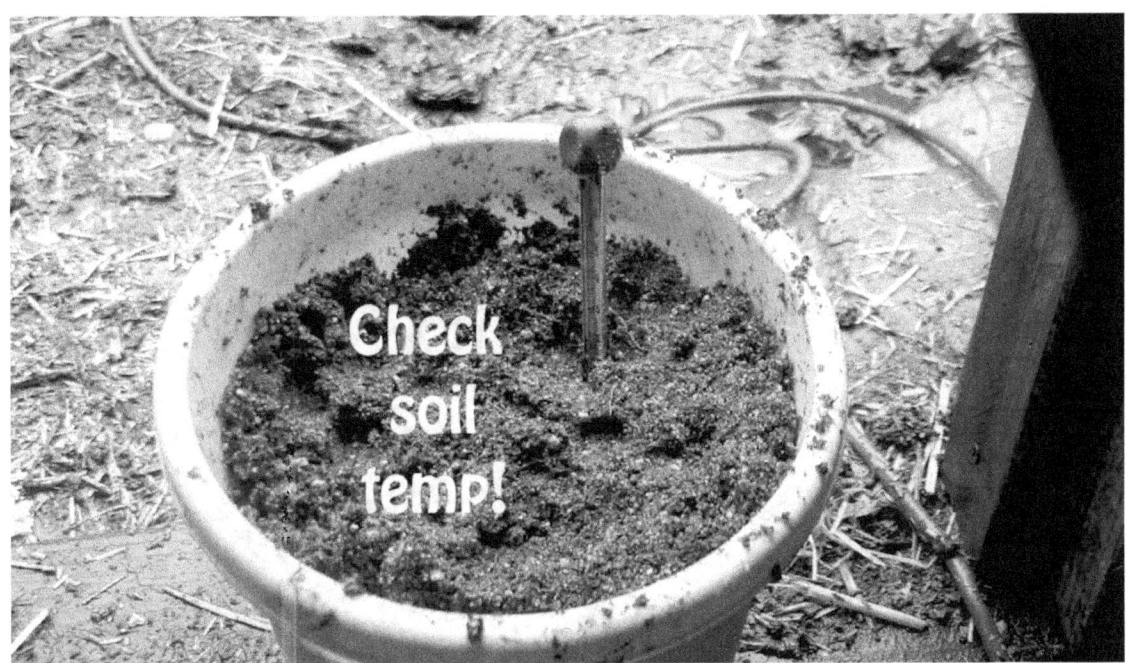

Before actually replanting your plant always check the soil temperature. Don't put a plant into freezing or super hot soil.

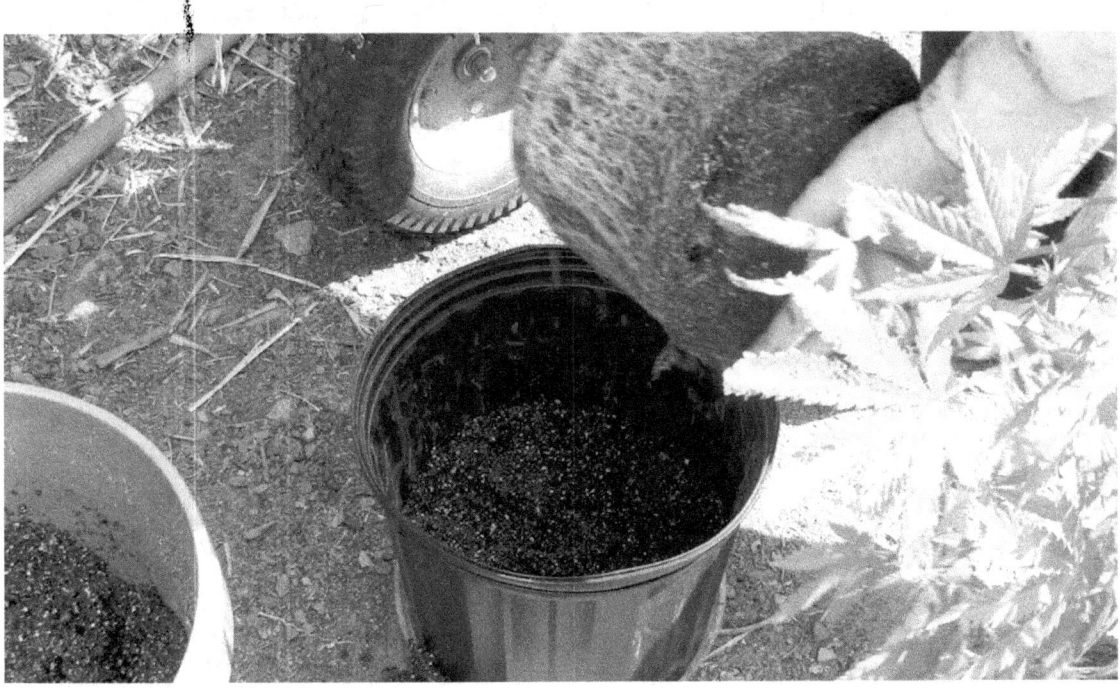

If replanting from a one gallon to three gallon or larger you may brush off the pebbles if you wish. You can see in the photo above that the roots have grown right to the edges the one gallon pot and that this plant is ready for repotting.

Do be careful when repotting not to brush the plants leaves against anything. In an earlier photo some abrasion damage was shown that was caused when I accidentally brushed the leaves of this plant against the ground.

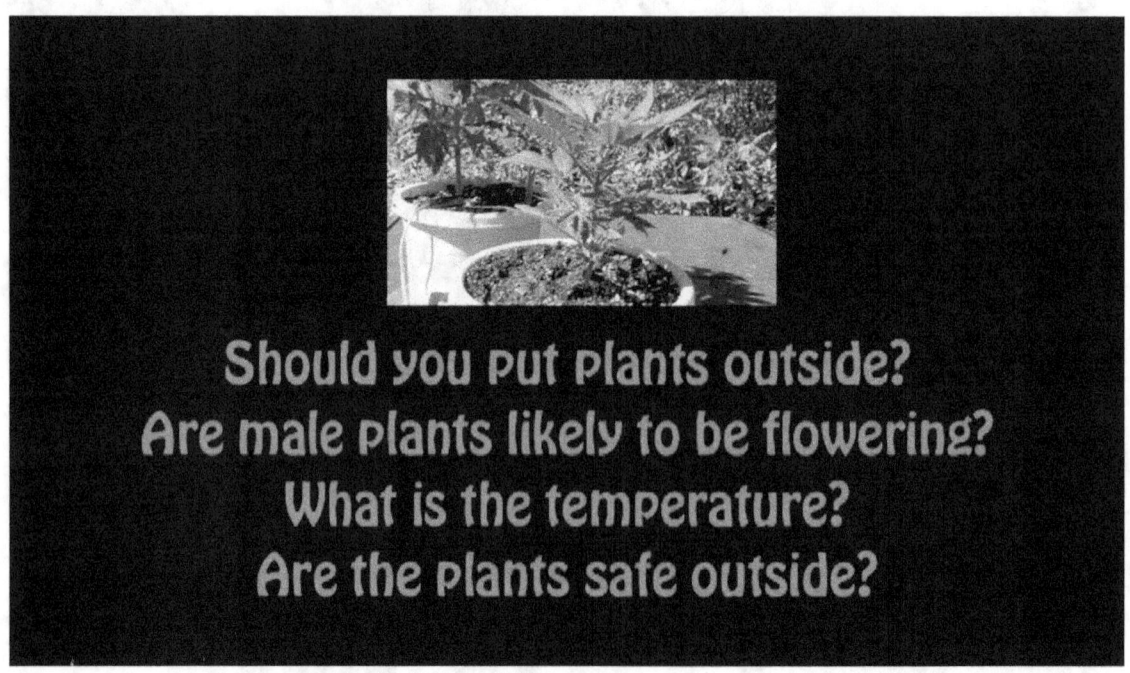

Should you put plants outside?
Are male plants likely to be flowering?
What is the temperature?
Are the plants safe outside?

In summer, if you have a safe place outside to put plants where they will get sunlight you can take advantage of the suns powerful rays. Questions you should ask before putting plants outside are:

o Are the plants safe?
o Could there be male plants flowering (giving off pollen) in the area?
o What is the temperature?   Does it get very cold at night? (Assuming you leave them out at night.) Or does the temperature get too hot in the sun. (Don't let the soil temp get higher than 85° F. If the temperature gets too hot use a screen of some sort to filter out the sun.
o Are there insects that could eat the plant or cause the spread of disease, or damage the plant in another way.

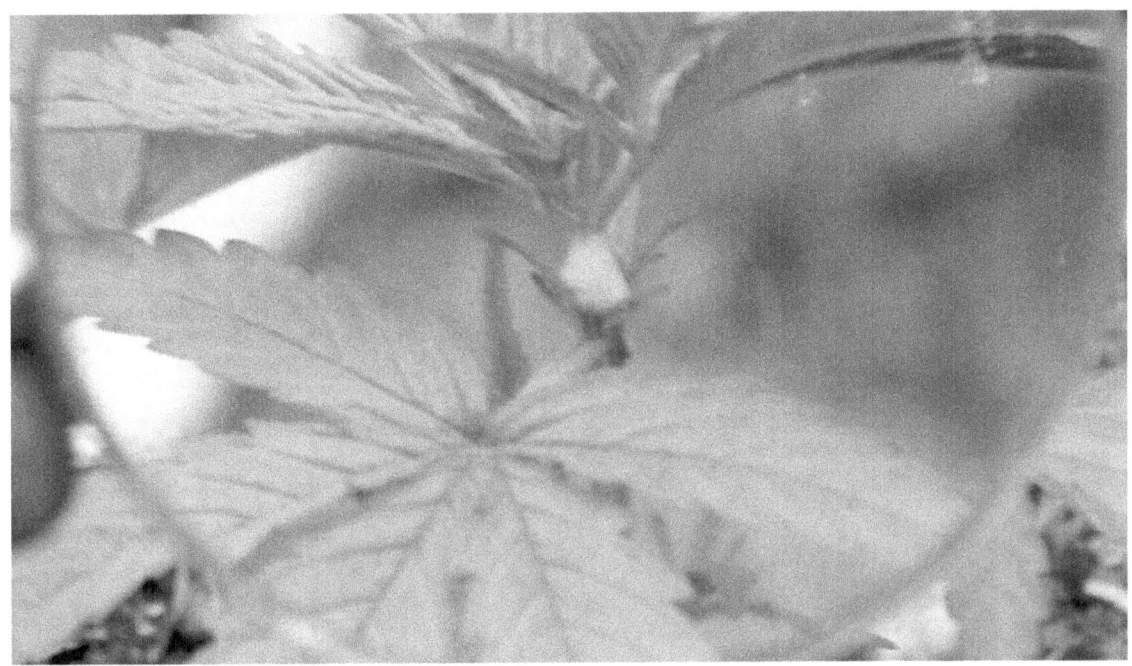

If you keep you plant indoors you should see very little in the way of insect problems. In fact, you should, with only 6 plants, never see an insect problem that you can't solve simply by picking the insects off.

The one plant I did have an insect (singular) problem was a male clone I had made before realizing the mother plant was male. As an experiment I put the plant outside. After it had been growing a month I found a small cluster of bubbles indicating a spittle bug. This bug is not fatal to marijuana, but will slow down growth.

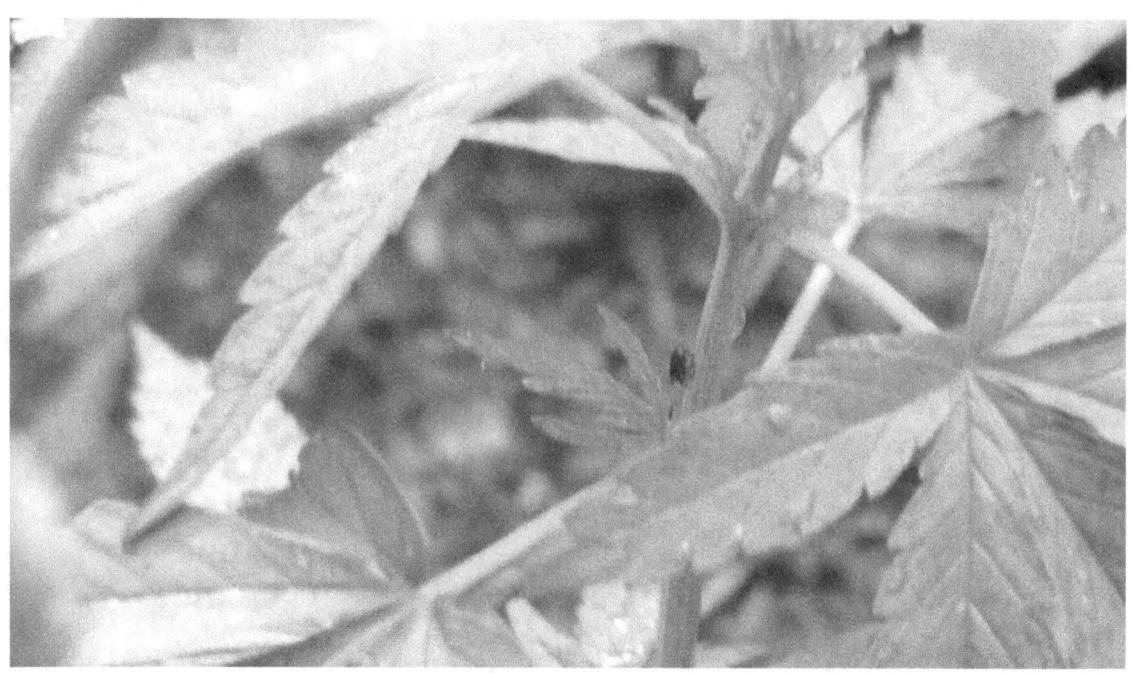

I sprayed the spittle with a .5% nitrosyme solution (just what I had on hand) and the spittle bug ran down the stem (you can see him in the above photo.) He recreated his spittle and I sprayed it again. This time when he ran down the plant he did not create more spittle. He, in fact, hung out on the plant, spittleless, until a deer ate the plant.

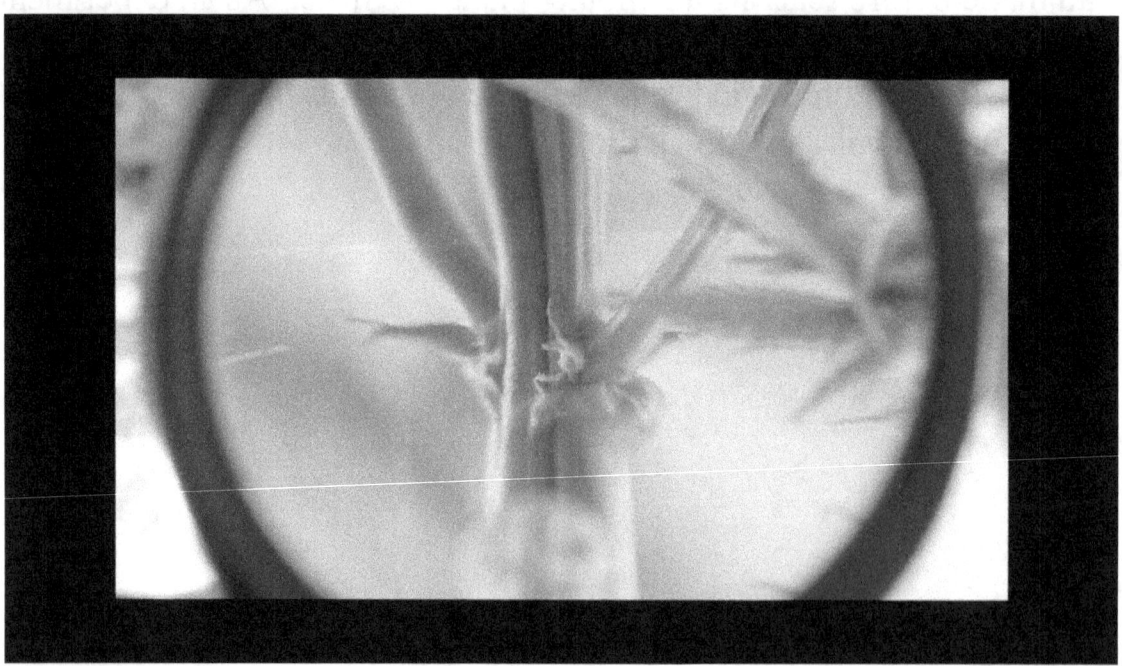

Once your plants show signs of sexual maturity, as does the female plant above, you can move the plants into the bloom shed, and put them on a 12 hours of light, 12 hours of complete darkness cycle. Remember that it is important the darkness be complete. Have someone shut you inside the shed to make sure the darkness is complete.   Going into the shed in the middle of the night will revert the plant to the growing phase.

I did, once, come back late one day and my blooming plant received 30 minutes of extra light. I kept the plant an extra 40 minutes in the dark the next day and there seemed to be no ill effect.

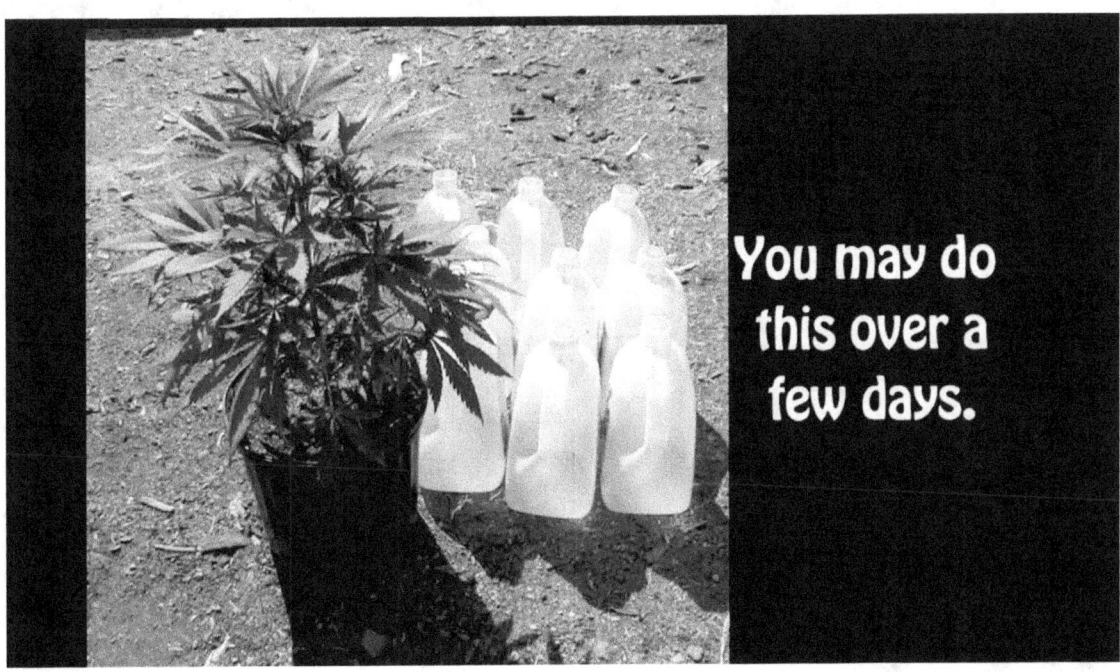

You may do this over a few days.

Before moving a plant to the bloom shed many people flush the pot with 3 times its volume of water. That is for a 3 gallon pot, as shown, you might use 9 gallons of water. This can take awhile so you might want to allow a day or two for the flushing.   The purpose is to remove the original fertilizer byproducts in the soil and prepare for the new blooming fertilizer you'll be using.

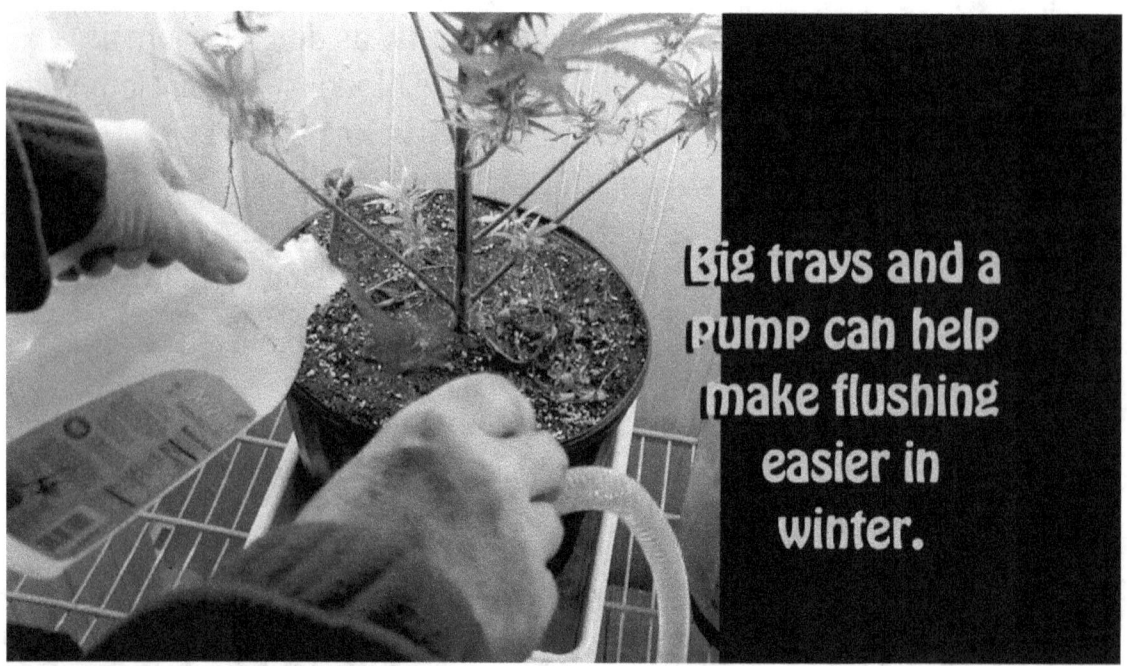

Big trays and a pump can help make flushing easier in winter.

A big tray to catch the water. In this case one I stole from a refrigerator, and a pump can make flushing easier in winter.

Just as I used ¼ strength Miracle Grow Organic for the growing stage I mixed a ¼ strength 0-10-10 mixture for my bloom fertilizer. I kept track of my mixtures in the back of my notebook.

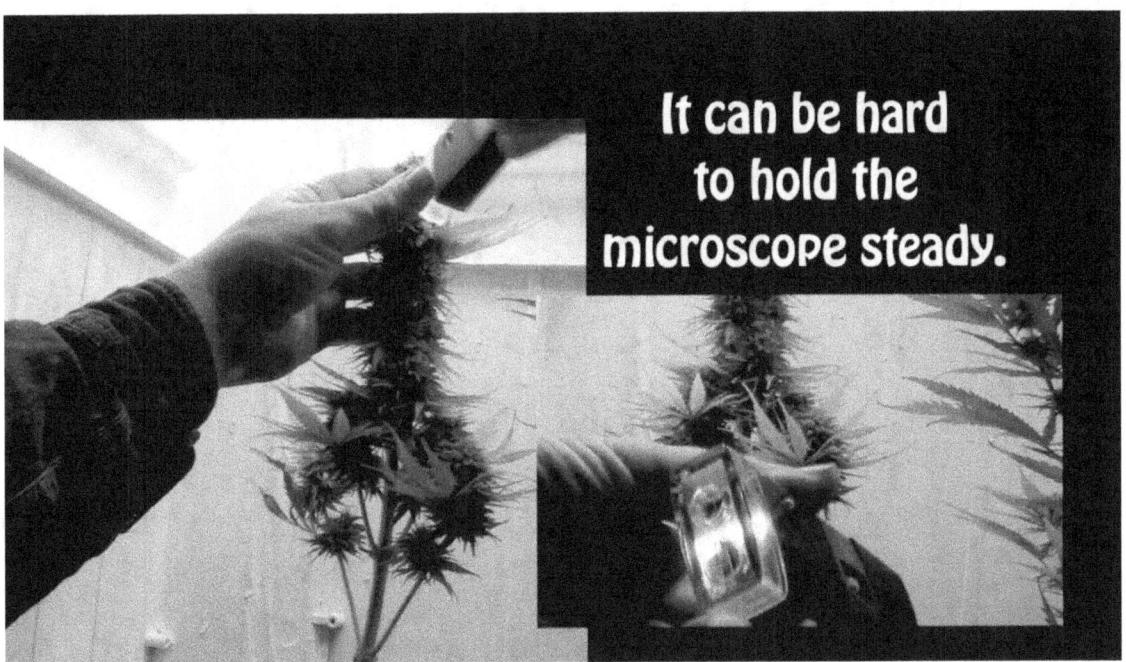

It can be hard to hold the microscope steady.

Information that came with your seed will give you some idea of how long the blooming process will take for your medicine. My iced grapefruit was listed as take 8 weeks to bloom. The nitrosyme, because it speeds up growth, reduced that to 7 weeks. But the only real way to tell if your plant is ready is with a handheld microscope or jeweler's loop. (Jeweler's loops are a little easier to use.) By examining the plant with your microscope you'll be able to see the tricomes, the resin glands on the buds.

Make sure that the microscope you buy has a light and if you have a hard time holding still enough to see you can try putting some bud in a bottle cap and placing the microscope across the top.

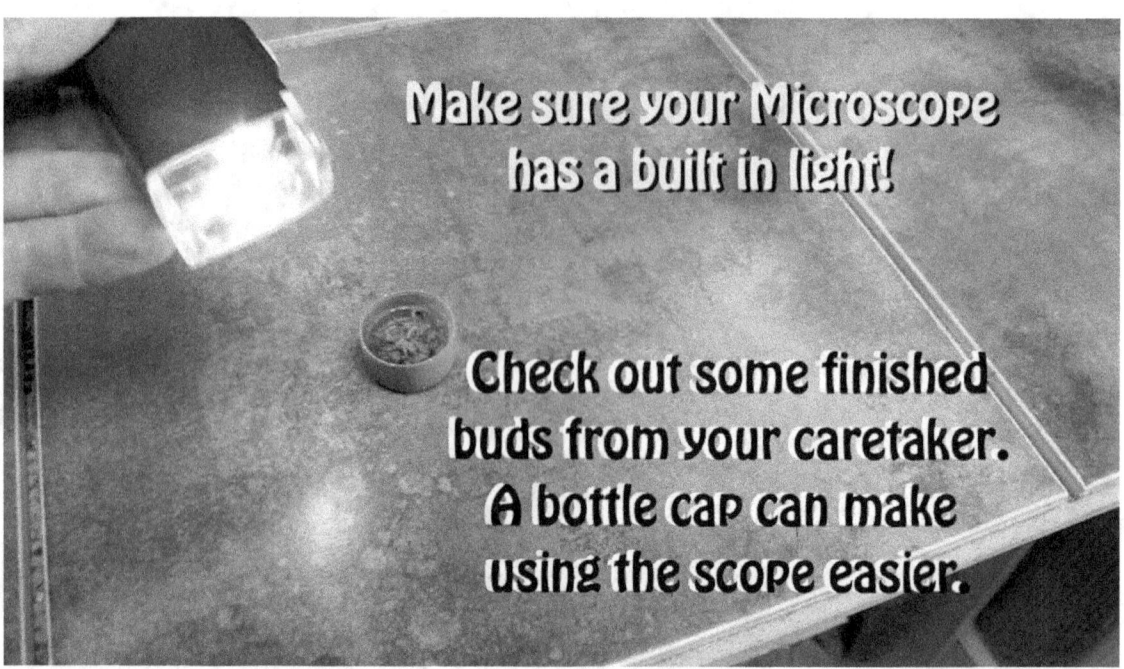

Make sure your Microscope has a built in light!

Check out some finished buds from your caretaker. A bottle cap can make using the scope easier.

Resin glands which look like an odd erect penis, start out clear and then become cloudy. Many people harvest when the glands turn milky and some prefer that the glands are in the next stage: turning amber.

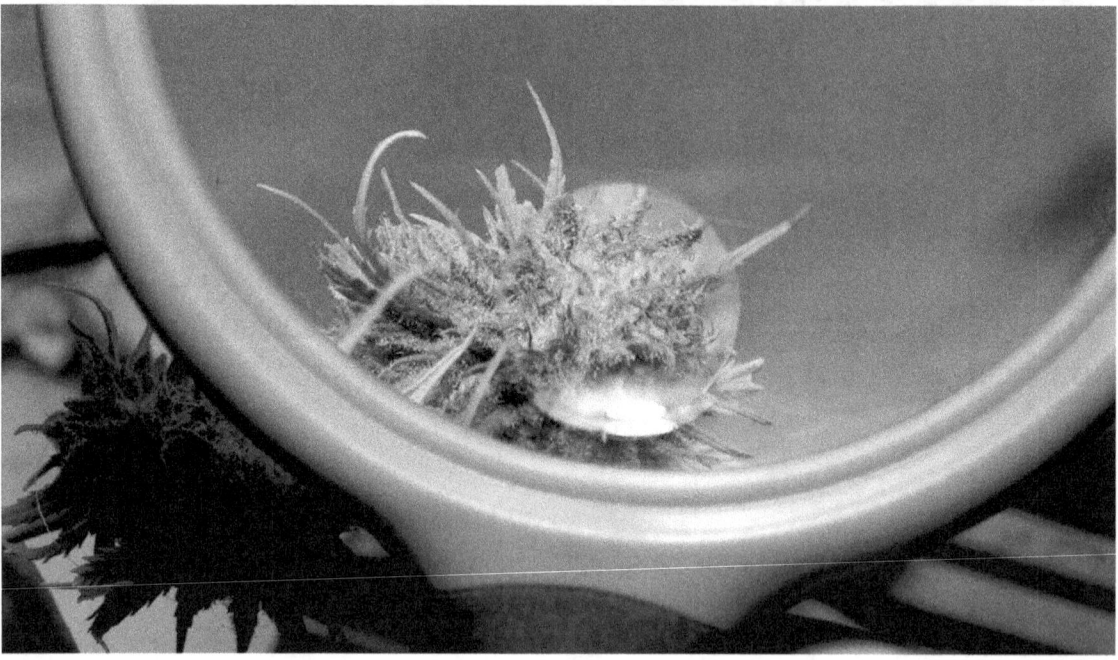

You can make out the glands with a big magnifying glass but to really see them you will need a jeweler's loop or microscope.

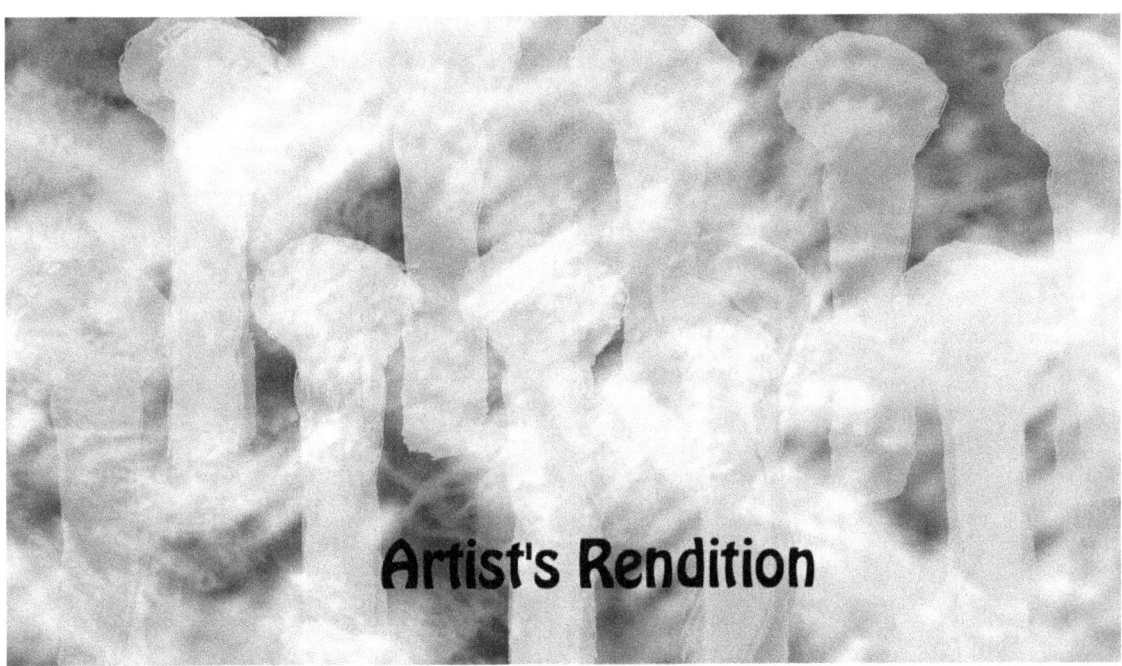

Artist's Rendition

Just before harvest, I do a few things to help keep a fertilizer flavor from getting into the plant and to increase resin. To reduce fertilizer taste I water with pure water for the last ten days of growth. To increase resin production I cover the plants for the last 36 hours with black plastic bags completely shutting out all light. This visible increased the resin on my buds.

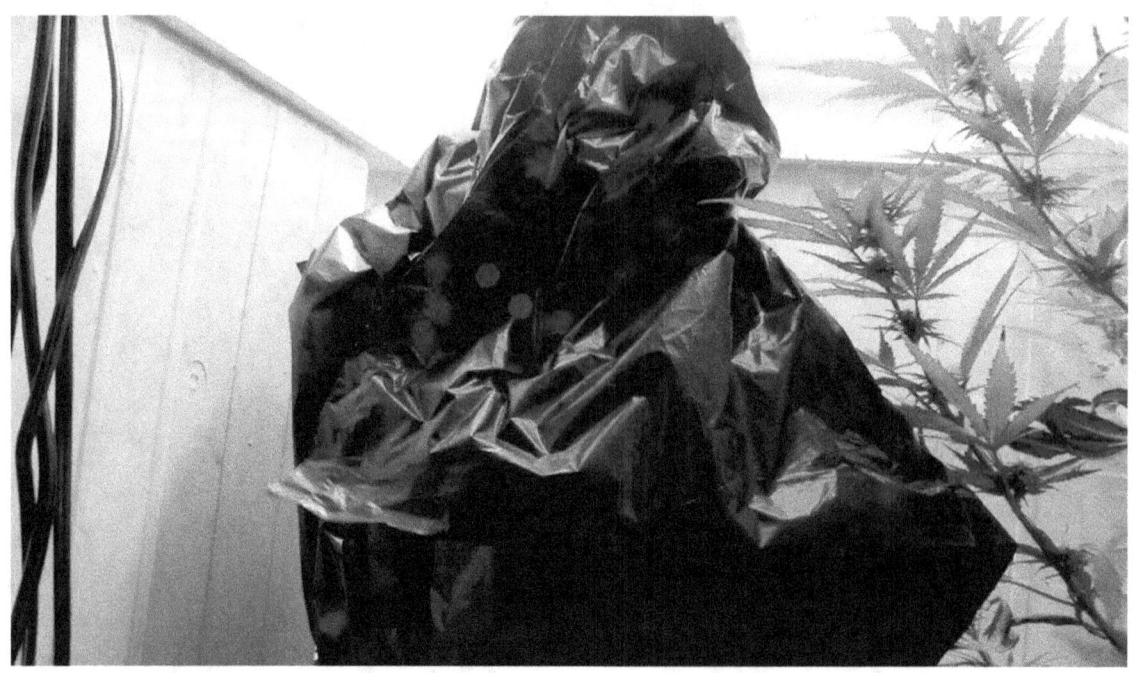

When the cover comes off it is time to harvest the buds.

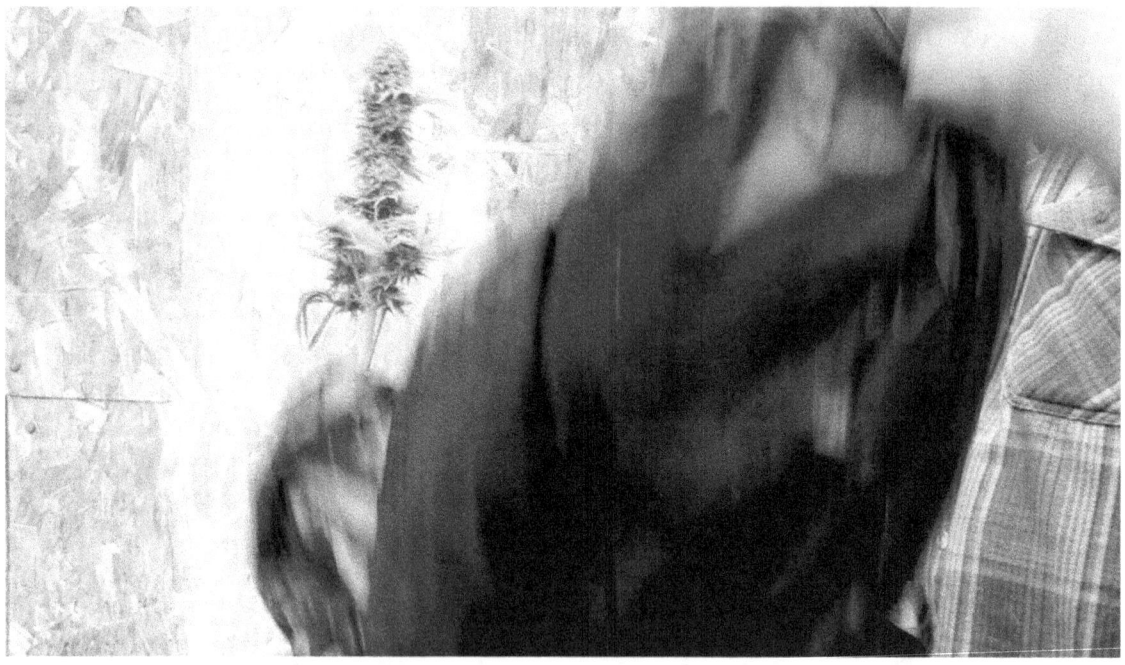

Since you are only growing for your own use there is no real need to trim the buds. And, in fact, if you are going to make butter or tincture you don't have to do anything with the leaves.

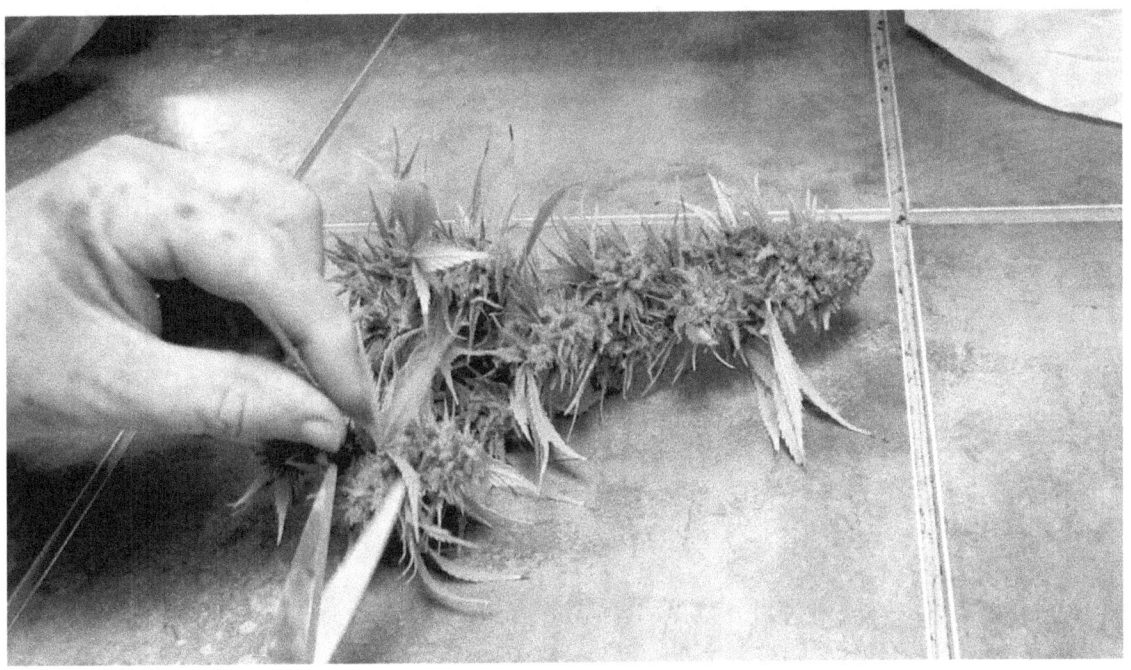

Just remove the largest leaves and hand the stem to dry inside a cardboard box with a hole in it for circulation.

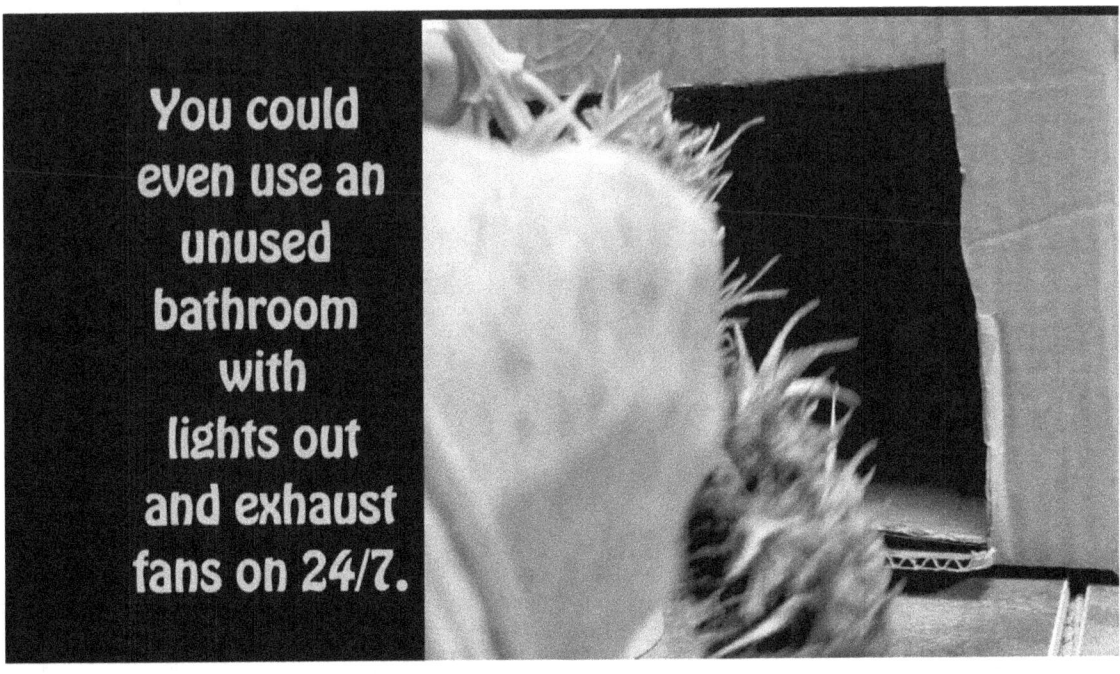

You could even use an unused bathroom with lights out and exhaust fans on 24/7.

I usually leave my plants in the box for about 5 days then move the almost dry buds to a mason jar for final curing.

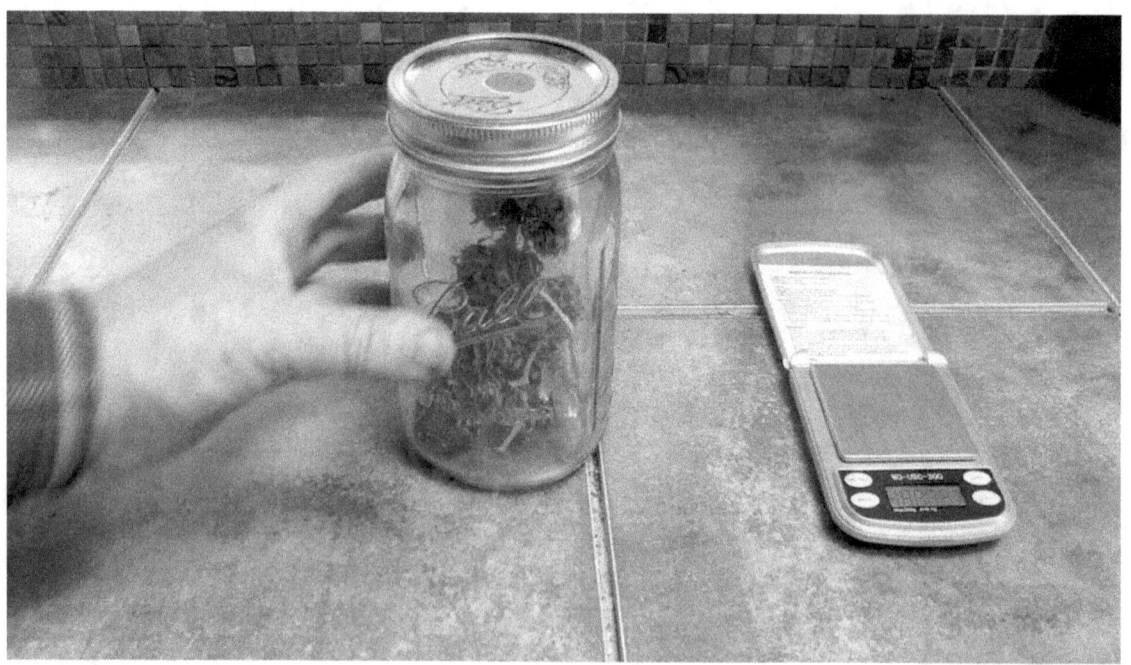

To finish up, just open the mason jar from time to time releasing more moisture. This will dry the plants and cure the resin.

And that's it. Good luck with your medicine.